Y0-BRC-305

Runaway #1 Bestseller!

Pure Fat Burning Fuel:
Follow This Simple, Heart Healthy Path To Total Fat Loss

Including 23 Delicious, Fat Melting, Full Color Recipes!

By #1 Bestselling Author:
Isabel De Los Rios

Visit www.MyFatBurningBonus.com And Get Your FREE Mouth Watering Recipes And More!

Discover What <u>Real Buyers</u> Of Pure Fat Burning Fuel Are Saying!

"Here she is again with another fantastic product! Since discovering Isabel and her program I have devoured everything she has written - it is all so sensible and straight forward. This latest product is another example of Isabel presenting thorough research in a user-friendly way. Thanks Isabel!" - Jessica

"I love, love, love Isabel and her ideas and suggestions. She is always down to earth and makes sure you understand HOW to do everything she suggests! I look forward to each new email from her and have used many of her tips!" - Suzy

"I have been a member of Beyond Diet for quite a while now but have just been "playing" with it. This book has simply fired me up to really give the plan my whole attention and effort. Thanks Isabel! Fantastic!" - Barbara Brenchley

"Isabel tells it like it is. Sugar in processed foods is the main culprit today. Type 2 Diabetes here we come. Please read this book and take heed!" - Remi Reader

"First healthy diet I have found that I could work with. Lost inches of fat right away and kept on losing it. I have lost 15 pounds so far and have more energy now than I have for a long time." - Carol Drennan

"I've been following Isabel for a couple years now, starting with her Diet Solution books - good information that she has fully researched and trying to point people in a direction on how to eat healthy for life; not only to lose weight but to improve overall health." - Mary Marino

"Wonderful book. Completely changes the way you think about food. Reeducates the lifetime dieter. Well worth the money. Thanks Isabel." - Fat Girl

"Great info for all to get healthy and not feel deprived!! Super easy to follow recipes. Looking forward to making some!" - Dana Stokes

"Feel better live longer with a satisfying way to enjoy the food that truly nourishes your body. I always have plenty of food at my main meals and I keep snacks for in between times. I lost 30 lbs. and feel great." - Edwardo

"Thank you for letting me know about the items in this book that I did not know about. I am excited to be able to use this information and to able to use it from now on to help me further lose my unwanted weight. The information is just what I needed thank you." - Karen Kimber

"I found Isabel's information about a year ago and was dedicated to follow her advice. I have gotten very similar advice from a functional medicine doctor previously, Isabel's book just made it easier. Now that she has this one out, I bought it as soon as it was available. I fell back into my sugar habit, and need to climb out of it again. i am motivated and the timing of this book couldn't be better for me." - Tooth Fairy

"You've done it again!! Took something complicated and broke it down to where we could understand it. Wonderful.....See you "lighter" LOL this was my first experience purchasing a book through Amazon, and it was easy!!! Thank you!!!!" - Karen H

"After just a cursory review, I'm sure this is going to be a great reference tool--and so slick! I really like the recipes and can't wait to view the videos." - Suki

"Not just a diet, but a healthy lifestyle. Really loved reading and implementing these guidelines into my life. Thank you for an excellent book!!" - Cindy Rogers

"I am trying so hard to eat healthy. It's been such a battle until I found Beyond Diet. Isabel has helped me learn how to shop and figure out exactly what I need to stay away from. I can't thank her enough. This new book makes it even easier." - Miss Patty

"I had read the book "Eat Fat to Lose Fat" several years ago. It was recommended to me by my naturopath. What a revelation! I am SO glad Isabel is spreading the good word about eating the proper fats to stay healthy. Eating radically less sugar is a tough transition for many of us, but eating the proper fats can make the change to a low/no sugar eating plan SO much easier. Hooray to Isabel for getting this information out in a straight forward, easy to understand way." - Rya Rugweaver

"Ok, here is my honest review. The content and concepts of this book really got my brain turning, and the online resources were fabulous. I really liked how fast of read it was and how once a point was made we were able to move on. The online videos were amazing, and really helped me when showing my husband some of the changes we will be having in our home now. My only complaint is it was a bit dry Isabel was fun and entertaining on in the online videos and I was not able to get that as much in the reading of this book." - Aubrey Jane

"This book made me pretty angry. I have been wasting a lot of time with the other diets and plans out there and the reasons Isabel gives for them not working makes PERFECT sense. My whole life all the doctors kept telling me to watch my fat intake. I kept feeling hungry all the time and ended up getting bigger and unhealthier. Thank goodness I found this book and found out about all the disinformation I was getting fed. I feel like I've wasted most of my life heading down the wrong road. Time to make some major changes. And this time it actually feels possible." - Cameron Williams

"Having been considered by doctors as "obese" since I was 16 this whole weight loss thing has been a major issue for me for a long time. What I truly relate to in this book is what she says about how the mainstream & diet industries have basically been making us fatter for decades. Every time my parents would take me to see the doctor, he would tell them "get him on a low fat diet, lots of whole grains, we've got to get his weight down.

It wasn't until roughly 2 years ago that I first heard about the problem with simple carbs and sugars and how the exact advice my doctors were giving me was the exact reason I kept gaining weight year after year.

What I really love about this book is that it hits home in some powerful ways. Isabel goes beyond just a "diet" and focuses more on the joys of eating the RIGHT foods. She wants you to focus more on being fully rather than starving yourself. The meal plans work, the science works, and the program just flat out works.

Since I've modified my eating habits, using the simple program she lays out, I've finally been able to start dropping fat. Clearly I'm not to my goal yet (I just started!) but for the FIRST TIME I'm actually seeing real progress and know it's possible to change.

This is a VERY solid book if you want to get rid of extra fat without health-harming, in effective crash diets." - S. Davis

"All I can say is "WOW!!!" I want to go back and read the whole thing again, as well as have everyone in my family read it!" - Skinny Vickie

"Beyond Diet is the most intelligent approach to not only lose fat, but to also just feel really healthy. After all you could be the wealthiest person in the world, but what good would it do if you were bedridden. This is your smartest option to feel your best even if you don't have a perfect body." - Lou

"This book is great! It's so helpful and easy to read and understand. Can't wait to use these helpful tips." - L.R.

"This is a great supplement to the materials I got on the Beyond Diet website. The information is well laid out and easy to read which makes it easier to understand and implement. Thanks!" - Tina M. Purvis

"Tell your friends and family that they don't have to diet. This book explains this simple fact. Education is our greatest tool." - Deb

"Great information on food to share with my own family. Eating healthy. On my way to a better, healthier, life and better yet losing fat." - Elizabeth

"Excellent info about health and healthy eating. I am looking forward to using this info for shopping and cooking. Thank you!" - Geo Study

"I have been following Isabel for a while now, and she does an awesome job of explaining her program so it's easy to understand. She also has an awesome Facebook page and a community called Beyond Diet that has so much information. I am slowly making changes that I know will benefit my whole family. This is SO worth your time to read. This is the program that makes the most sense of anything I've read. Thanks Isabel!" - Liza Jane

"Isabel has helped me learn so much about eating healthy that I didn't know. I loved learning that it is not about depriving yourself that helps you lose weight but about making the right choices! I was surprised to learn some of the foods I thought were an absolute no no, are not only okay to eat but necessary for your health. This book has changed my thinking about eating healthy." - Rhonda Burket

"This book makes so much sense! Very very helpful and I'm ready to learn a new way of doing things. Life changing." Healthy For Life

"This plan is going to change my life. I believe in it already and can't wait to start. Everything I have read tells me this is a sustainable eating plan and I can't wait to empty my cupboards of rubbish and get down to the supermarket and health store ASAP." - Man Ian

"The information that Isabel covers in this book is easy to follow and is packed fully of information. She has really done her research and cares about your health. I would recommend this book to everyone I know! Thanks Isabel!!" - Student

"I just read through Pure Fat Burning Fuel and am so excited to finally have the knowledge I need to treat my body right! It is good to correct the confusing messages we get from so many sources!" - Heidi Dow

"Full of point on information! Isabel has done a wonderful job of explaining why we gain weight and how to lose it in a pure and healthy NATURAL way. This book combined with her Web Site is one powerful tool." - R Ruehl

"BD has changed the way I eat and is not a diet but a way of life. With all the chemicals in the food we eat and the air we breathe it's a wonder the obesity level isn't even higher. I have always said everything they put in our food is what is causing this epidemic." - Kimberly

"I am a member of beyond diet and have the diet solution program (dsp) eBook. Pure fat burning fuel looks very similar the dsp book but with up to date info and new recipes. Definitely a good book to add to your collection. Great price too!" - Luscious

"I read the information contained in this book about 18 months ago and lost 22% body fat and 45 pounds. It helped with my depression and changed my life-- I am no longer considered overweight or at risk for diabetes, no longer pre-hypertensive, no longer have high cholesterol, no longer have high triglycerides, I don't get sick nearly as much and even rarely have to use an inhaler for my asthma. If enough people ate like this the food industry would have to change to compete for our business-- they would have to offer healthier products. Get this and live this-- you will thank yourself!" - East Bay Dave

"I love Isabel and all of her great, practical advice. I can't wait to try these menus and her concept out. It doesn't look like I'll be food deprived or hungry at all!" - Kimber

"Thanks Isabel, I look forward to finishing your new book and using it along with the Beyond Diet information. I'm confident that it will be very helpful in getting any newbies started on the right path to healthy eating and a healthy lifestyle. Bon Appetite!" - W Bunny

"I really agreed with a lot of the things that were said. I have tried dropping and avoiding fat and it did work so I'm going to try Isabel's way." - Try Again 20

"Isabel makes Beyond Diet easily understood. With the recipes included, it really sounds doable. I want to give it a try!" - JST

"I just received the book and am finding it very informative. I am learning what makes me fat and what I can do about it without the feared dieting routine. I am looking foward to using her eating plan. Thank you so much." - Lois M

"As Brad's wife, I have been a fan of Isabel De Los Rios since the Beyond Diet days! She has never lead me wrong, and I totally agree with her philosophy on healthy eating. Can't wait to finish the book...from what I've read so far, it's a winner!" - Brad Simon

"Isabel has written the best lifelong eating plan I have seen. She is very balanced and has great information to share. Her plan is obtainable and easy to follow." - Victoria

"The money-saving and tips on shopping are extremely helpful. I also really love the meal plans. Isabel has been there and really knows how being overweight feels." - Purple Girl Mary

"After looking through the plan, it seems like it is very doable. It's very common sense with no weird funky schedules to follow. The recipes look and sound yummy. The grocery shopping lists are a plus. Everything is explained so well." - K Wagner

Contents

Welcome To Your New Life!

Let's start with a story. It goes like this: "There once was a girl who was fat. Then she wasn't. She became lean and toned and loved life. The end."

Obnoxious, right? Doesn't it seem way too simple? Like it's never going to happen for you in a million years? If you're reading this, you're probably struggling with weight loss. I hope you've enjoyed that struggle, because that part of your life ends now.

Right now, you're probably in the same place that I was a few years ago: overweight, tired, and uncomfortable in my clothes. I would guess that you identify with more than a few of the following descriptions:

- You've read and tried every diet book, diet pill, and supplement known to mankind.

- Your personal collection of exercise VHS videos and DVDs is large enough that you could open your own Blockbuster or Netflix.

- You've tried numerous gyms and personal trainers, but nothing seemed to work.

- You've tried starving yourself to become skinny.

- Your attempts to lose weight result in you feeling hungry all the time.

- You feel like you have no energy.

- You've felt the embarrassing stress of failing yet another diet plan and asked yourself: *What am I doing wrong?*

Despite your best efforts - and we're talking *years* of your best efforts - do you feel like you have nothing to show for it? Or perhaps you were one of the lucky ones that managed to get some results. Maybe you looked and felt better for a month or so. But then your weight suddenly and mysteriously ballooned back to its original level. I know what you're going through. I didn't always look like the girl you see on the cover. I used to be pretty heavy.

The story from the beginning of the book is mine. Granted it took a bit of doing, but rapid and lifelong weight loss can be simple. My story can be your story too. In the following pages, I'm going to share how I was able to achieve my personal weight loss goals and transform into that other, far more amazing picture.

Guess what? I did it without hunger or dieting. I don't limit myself to nuts and berries. I eat a lot - emphasis on *a lot* - of the delicious food I love, and it keeps me looking toned, lean, and full of energy.

In the next few sections I'm going to break down how this happened, why it hasn't happened for you yet, and how you will begin to see rapid weight loss results through this simple, real world program. No matter how you may feel right now, what solutions you may have tried in the past, or how many times you may have played with the diet yo-yo, there is one fact you must remember: *It's not your fault and you are not alone.* Being overweight is one of the greatest social and economic stigmas that can plague an individual. I felt it every day of my life. On the upside, it's not a lonely group. Worldwide, almost 1.5 billion adults are classified as overweight or obese. Nearly seventy percent of the American population is currently overweight. And despite the fact that the percentage of obese people attempting to lose weight is increasing, the rate of obesity is continually on the rise. So where is everyone going wrong? What's wrong is until recently nearly every source of "health advice" was actually dishing out a recipe for obesity! (More on this in just a second.)

A large factor in the rate of obesity and its related diseases is the wealth of fallacious misinformation that was published decades ago and is still followed today. Some of the "healthy" eating habits that we follow religiously are actually contributing to obesity, and preventing us from succeeding in our weight loss goals.

Before we get started, you probably want to know who's dishing out the advice here, right?

In many ways I'm a lot like you. I've been overweight, I've been depressed, I've been out of hope. After I discovered what I'm about to share with you I was able to transform my entire body and health VERY quickly and have never looked back. Now I'm on a mission to solve this obesity epidemic once and for all. To date these shockingly simple and effective health boosting techniques have reached over 250,000 people. That number is growing every day.

I am the mother of two sweet boys and the wife of one of the best guys you'll ever meet. I graduated from Rutgers University with a degree in exercise physiology (a pre-med curriculum). As a Certified Strength and

Conditioning Specialist, I hold the highest and most advanced certification given by the National Strength and Conditioning Association. I am a Holistic Nutrition Lifestyle Coach, certified by the Corrective Holistic Exercise Kinesiology (C.H.E.K.) Institute in San Diego, California. I counsel many special populations, including diabetics, heart disease patients, cancer survivors, overweight individuals, and healthy individuals who wish to maintain health and prevent disease.[19]

I found my passion for nutrition as a teenager. The overweight daughter and granddaughter of type 2 diabetics, I was told that I was doomed to suffer from the same health problems as the generations preceding me. Not willing to sit around waiting for this grim prediction to become a reality, I studied every nutrition and diet book available in search of the answers to my family's weight and health problems. This led me to personally seek out doctors and health professionals that were using nutrition to get great results (as far as health and weight loss) with their patients and clients.[19]

I care because I've been there. I know what it feels like to look in the mirror and be completely unhappy with who is staring right back at you. I know what it feels like to want to wear certain clothes and feel good about the way you look. I don't want you to suffer like that. I don't want that for anybody.

Now let me tell you how I discovered the dietary secrets outlined in this book. Designing *Pure Fat Burning Fuel* was a bit of a lengthy process, and some of it was trial and error where I served as the human guinea pig. A lot of it was from my research. This combination is going to give you all the answers you seek. Here's a sneak peak at what is heading your way:

Part #1: How I finally lost tons of fat by kicking the "dieting." I used delicious foods, while never being hungry. This differs from what most diet plans preach.

Part #2: 5 Simple and extremely effective principles that are going to help you drop all the fat you want and keep it off for good. Say good bye to yo-yo dieting.

Part #3: The delicious fat burning meal plans and recipes to use to start losing fat right now.

Why Are So Many People Struggling With Weight Loss Anyway?

Have you every looked at photographs of Americans taken thirty to fifty years ago? It's hard to spot anyone that's overweight and both the men and women pictured resemble what would almost be seen today as modern supermodels.

By looking at their bodies, you'd think every single person was getting up at 4 in the morning to crank out a grueling two-hour workout. However, "working out" wasn't commonplace until later in the 20th century. Deliberate exercise was scarce during these times. Furthermore, the average American was no stranger to red meat. So how the heck were most Americans able to live and eat the way they did without thinking about their waist lines?

The reason so many people have become overweight in the past several decades is that we have been fed scientifically incorrect information about what constitutes "healthy" diets, and what kinds of foods are "good" and "bad." In order to lose weight, it is necessary to learn what kinds of foods your body needs to lose weight and remain healthy.

Paleolithic Chic: What Did Our Ancient Ancestors Eat?

Humans evolved somewhere between 2.6 million and 10,000 years ago - we won't go into the details of the exact timeline in this book. For our purposes, the important thing is that our Paleolithic ancestors ate quite differently. Their diet was the product of necessity: all food had to be either gathered from vegetation or hunted in the wild.

Historical and archaeological evidence shows hunter-gatherers tended to be lean, healthy, and mostly free from signs and symptoms of chronic diseases. Our Paleolithic ancestors had to exert themselves every single day to obtain food, water, and protection. Hunter-gatherers walked five to ten miles daily as they foraged and hunted for food, and staying alive meant lifting, carrying, running, climbing, stretching and leaping, and they therefore avoided weight gain even in times of abundance. Days of heavy exertion were followed by recover days. In modern terms, these people cross-trained with aerobic, resistance, and flexibility exercises. According to recent data on physical activity, fitness programs that use various exercises are the most effective in preventing cardiovascular diseases.[1]

The hunter-gatherer way of life continued through the early stages of Westernization. However, people began to migrate from farming communities to urban areas between 1750 and 1900 AD. As the population began to boom and the number of farmers available to meet the food demand continued to decrease, the agricultural focus shifted from quality to quantity. Corn and wheat emerged as easy and cheap crops to produce, and grains began to replace vegetables as the foundation of our diet.[2]

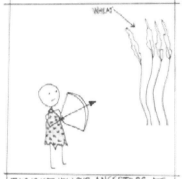

As hunter-gatherer societies changed to agricultural grain-based diets, overall health deteriorated. Average adult height was considerably shorter for both men and women who ate cereals and starches, compared to their hunter-gatherer ancestors who consumed lean meats, fruits, and vegetables. In addition, studies of bones and teeth reveal that populations who changed to a grain-based diet had shorter life spans, higher childhood mortality, and a higher incidence of osteoporosis, rickets, and various other mineral- and vitamin-deficiency diseases.[3]

When these people adopt western diets, their health declines and they begin to exhibit signs and symptoms of "diseases of civilization," such as obesity, type 2 diabetes, and atherosclerosis. Today, people tend to live in mechanical urban environments, living mostly sedentary lives and eating a highly processed artificial diet. As a result, two-thirds of Americans are overweight or obese. The lifetime occurrence of hypertension is at an astonishing ninety percent, and forty percent of middle-aged American adults have metabolic syndrome.[4]

Cardiovascular disease accounts for forty-one percent of all fatalities and remains the number one cause of death in America.[5] The prevalence of heart disease in the United States is projected to double during the next fifty years. Despite astounding pharmacological and technological advances, the epidemic of cardiovascular disease continues.[6] Meanwhile, elderly people in modern hunter-gatherer societies have been shown to be generally free of the signs and symptoms of chronic diseases such as obesity, high blood pressure, and high cholesterol, which commonly afflict the elderly in Western societies.[7] Although it is certainly true that the average person's lifespan in one such society is not as long as the average lifespan in modern America, this is due to the accidents and traumas associated with living largely in the elements and without modern medicine, and is not the consequence of widespread chronic degenerative diseases.[8]

What we need to remember is that we are all still these same hunters and gatherers from thousands of years ago. The fact is that our lifestyle has radically changed, but our overall genetic makeup has basically stayed the same. A fundamental axiom of biology holds that living things do best in the environment and on the diet for which they were genetically adapted.[9] Our ancestors lived off fresh meats, leaves, and roots - foods that promote good health and are high in beneficial nutrients such as soluble fiber, antioxidant vitamins, phytochemicals, Omega-3 and monounsaturated fats, and low-glycemic carbohydrates. The standard American diet today consists mostly of refined sugars and grains, saturated and trans fats, salt, high-glycemic carbohydrates, and processed foods.[10] Consequently, we have billions of people with the same nutritional requirements as they did thousands of years ago consuming a diet that they are not genetically able to tolerate. Furthermore, we are genetically programmed to live an extremely active lifestyle, but most of us live a sedentary life. This makes us vulnerable to obesity, hypertension, metabolic syndrome, diabetes, and most types of cardiovascular disease.[11]

In order to reduce widespread obesity and the occurrence of chronic degenerative diseases, we need to adjust our current non-adaptive diet and lifestyle to mimic the milieu for which we are genetically designed. Luckily for us, we are the first generation to have the genetic and scientific knowledge to allow us to recreate this lifestyle. We can analyze what foods are necessary to keep the body healthy and lean and understand why it works. The focus of this book is adjusting our diets, but please keep in mind that regular exercise is crucial to maintaining a healthy body too. Although exercise is now an option rather than a requirement for survival, it is still important to exercise as though your life depends on it - in a way, it still does.[12]

Why Am I Having Trouble Losing Weight?

Early in my career, I was working as a personal trainer in New Jersey at a private studio with five other trainers. Most of us stuck to the same basic mantra: *Eat healthy, exercise regularly, lose weight.* However, this basic advice didn't work for all of us. In particular, it didn't work for *me*.

One of the other trainers, "Joe," was a bit of a wise guy. In the beginning, I wasn't a huge fan of his arrogant attitude. One conversation with Joe went something like this:

> *Joe: Isabel, what's up with the same breakfast every day? Doesn't that get boring?*
>
> *Me: Who cares? I need to get this fat off my legs, so I'll do what it takes.*
>
> *Joe: That's funny. Egg whites and whole wheat bread will make you fatter. Good luck with that.*

Right about here, I hate Joe. But just because I'm a glutton for punishment, I ask him to elaborate.

> *Me: Please, Joe. Enlighten me with your theories. Should I be eating bacon instead? Maybe that would make me lose weight?*
>
> *I laughed exaggeratedly.*
>
> *Joe: Actually, you are one hundred percent correct. If you ate bacon instead of what you're eating now, you probably would lose a ton of weight.*
>
> *Me: Listen, Joe. I'm not going on the Atkins diet. That is just crazy and I know a lot of people who've gotten sick eating tons of bacon and cheese so I don't buy it.*
>
> *Joe: Okay. So be fat.*

Did I mention he was obnoxious?

I really didn't engage much with Joe after that, but I did overhear him talking to his clients. I heard pearls of wisdom along the lines of, *"Stop drinking Crystal Light. It's making you fat,"* or *"Why in the world would you ever think being a vegetarian would make you lose weight?"* Other notable lines included, *"Why are you snacking on fruit? You'll never lose weight like that,"* and *"You want to go out Saturday night?"* I guess he wasn't obnoxious to everyone.

Basically, it seemed that good ole Joe was always doing just the opposite of what everyone else was doing: slathering butter on his food, eating whole egg omelets, and consuming more food in one day than most small villages. Obviously, my first assumption was that he was one of those genetically fatless robots with superhuman metabolisms, one that wouldn't even slow down after the age of thirty. However, Joe always carried around his "fat" pictures with him, so I knew that he was not naturally lean or born with perfect genes. So I swallowed my pride and finally asked Joe what the deal was.

"Isabel," he said, "I'm going to tell you the one thing you need to know, and you'll be able to easily lose all the weight you want and still eat delicious food."

Sounds a lot like the too-simple story from the beginning of this book, doesn't it? But as much as I hate to admit it, obnoxious butter-eating Joe was right. The common approach to weight loss was all wrong. The dialogue about how to lose weight involves a lot of misinformation.

5 Shockingly Common Mistakes Almost Nobody Knows About That Are Keeping You Fat

Common Mistake #1: Restricting caloric intake in an attempt to lose weight.

Sure, this may work for a very short time, but once hunger strikes it becomes really difficult to eat like a bird and still enjoy life. Eat foods that keep your body burning fuel all day long, and you'll never have to worry about counting another calorie again. This book focuses on eating the right kind of foods, and I will walk you step-by-step through the process of restructuring the way you think about "good" and "bad" foods.

Common Mistake #2: Avoiding fat, especially saturated fat, in order to lose inches.

Are you ready for what I'm about to say? Eat a ton of saturated fat in order to be the healthiest and leanest you've ever been. Did you fall out of your chair? It's true: Eating a ton of saturated fat is going to be the best strategy you implement towards a lean body and a healthy heart.

Common Mistake #3: Thinking you have to go on a "diet" to lose weight.

We've all fallen for fad diets. We've all started off on a new and promising eating program, dutifully eating cardboard-flavored everything and ignoring our body's cravings. The first few days go pretty well, and you can handle how hungry you feel. But by the end of the first week you are craving so much "bad" food that it's all you think about.

Forget the word "diet"—wipe it from your vocabulary. "Dieting" suggests lumping all the foods you like to eat in one category and promising that you'll never ever eat them again, which is why dieting so often ends in relapse. Pure Fat Burning Fuel teaches you how to restructure the way you think about food so that you can continue to eat delicious food. It emphasizes losing weight in an enjoyable way, allowing you to go on with your life, do the things you enjoy doing...and forget about dieting. As we'll discuss soon, your body usually craves the foods it needs to be healthy. The trick is to learn which foods to eat and which to avoid so that your body is getting what it needs.

Common Mistake #4: Following a cookie cutter meal plan that is not designed for your body.

Weight-loss is not meant to be "one size fits all." You're different than everyone else, so why would you go on the same diet as everyone else? We all have unique bodies with unique needs, and in order to change your body, you have to focus on its unique chemistry. Don't compare your weight loss program to your sister's or best friend's or boss', because the key to healthy weight loss is a plan that fulfills your body's needs.

Common Mistake #5: Eating food labeled low-fat, low-carb, or heart healthy.

This is one of the biggest ways to sabotage your weight-loss. If you're eating food that is low-fat or low-carb, your taste buds probably aren't happy. Unhappy taste buds lead to cravings, and cravings lead to relapse. Fat curbs your hunger and cravings, and less fat means that you'll be tempted to eat more reduced-fat food because you're feeling unsatisfied. Fat-free and reduced-fat versions of food usually contain more sugar and salt than full fat versions, because removing fat means that taste needs to be put back in somehow.

> *"From age 40 to 50 I counted calories (had to keep under 1100 cal/ day to lose weight) and exercised. I lost 7 lbs once a year between January and April and spent the rest of the year adding them on again. This was clearly not working and not a long-term strategy at all. After 2 months on the BD program, I started getting more energy and feeling less body pains. My self-confidence has improved now that I feel more representable. I have fun developing recipes and I have never enjoyed cooking so much in my life! I have lived very alone for the last 6 years, but after answering BD questions and connected with people that way I have started making friends outside the house too." - Vera H. Olcott, Oxford, OH*

Sculpting Your Dream Body & Ideal Well-being

If you had a magic wand, and could make any wish come true, what would you ask for in terms of your weight, your body, and your health?

Don't hold back. Really think about it. I'm letting you use my very precious and extremely effective magic wand. Don't miss out on the opportunity.

I want you to really take some time to write down exactly how you want to look, exactly how you want to feel, and exactly how you want to fit into your clothes. If you want to jot down a few of the incredible compliments you're going to get on that hot body of yours, please do.

This exercise is how I got started, and I can remember doing it like it happened yesterday. I was visiting my parents for the weekend, up bright and early at 5 in the morning. I sat down at the dining table and I wrote exactly what I wanted to achieve in terms of my body. I understand this isn't the easiest thing to do, and people often dismiss this exercise as a waste of time and skip it. I can assure you that once you put it down in ink, you make it real.

If you're having trouble getting started, try beginning with some of the following questions:

#1: How much do you want to lose, and in what time frame? Example answer: I want to lose ten pounds in six weeks and fit into those old jeans from college. (Notice I didn't just write down "I want to lose weight." That would be too vague, and it's important to include lots of details.)

#2: How will you feel on the day you achieve your goal? Example answer: I haven't felt this great in years. My pants not only fit great, but I look amazing in them. And my spouse can't stop congratulating me on my progress. Man I look good! (This is the one where you really let the pen just flow.)

Before you move on to the next section, take a moment to write down your goals, using vivid and specific details. Make them come alive with emotion, feelings, and a description of exactly how you will feel on the day you have achieved this goal.

The Three Healthy Eating Tricks To Help You Melt Fat Quickly, Effectively And Permanently

The most overwhelming part about losing weight can be sorting through the science, medical facts, and technical jargon that accompanies many diet plans. As your coach and nutritionist, it is my job to decipher this information and give you the most important facts you need in a way that is easy to understand.

Losing weight means learning more about what you're eating and restructuring what you consider to be "good" and "bad" food. Weight loss is a huge industry and focus of study, meaning that there is inevitably a lot of misinformation passing as fact—even from reputable sources like doctors and respected dieticians. Therefore, before we break down *Pure Fat Burning Fuel* step-by-step, we need to discuss what "good" foods are and why they are good for you, and what "bad" foods are and why they're bad for you.

Keep in mind that the foundation of my program lies in the wisdom of Mother Nature. Just like the diet of our Paleolithic ancestors, our *Pure Fat Burning Fuel* eating plan is nutrient-dense and involves only nourishing, real foods in their whole food forms. Fortified and altered versions of food are inferior to real food because they have been stripped of their nutrients and injected with fattening preservatives and other ingredients (think real egg yolks vs. EggBeaters).

#1: Eat Protein in Every Meal

The Misconception: You've probably heard it before: "Too much protein damages your kidneys." Protein is comprised of amino acids, which are the building blocks that help us rebuild and repair muscles. The kidneys filter out unused amino acids as waste. Opponents of high protein diets often cite studies that seem to link protein consumption to impaired kidney function. For instance, the March 2003 edition of *Annals of Internal Medicine* published an 11-year study wherein researchers determined that out of 1,624 women with mild kidney problems, those who ate a high-protein diet experienced a faster rate of declining kidney function than those who did not.

The Truth: High-protein diets do not cause damage to people with healthy renal function. The above study demonstrates that high-protein consumption can be harmful to those who already have mild kidney damage. In fact, a study in the *International Journal of Obesity* comparing a high-protein weight-loss diet to a low-protein weight-loss diet concluded that healthy kidneys adapted to the increased protein intake and did not suffer any adverse effects. In your consideration of this issue, make note of the example set by professional athletes. If high-protein diets truly caused kidney failure, there would be a higher-than-normal rate of kidney disease among professional athletes, and this is simply not the case.

The Plan: There is no need to fear protein. Eating protein with every meal is a great way to stabilize your blood sugar, curb your hunger cravings, and boost glucagon levels—the fat burning hormone released by protein.

#2: Eat the Right Carbohydrates

The Misconception: Americans have become fearful of carbohydrates. We often hear that all carbohydrates are bad and will cause weight gain and increase body fat. For most people, the word "carbs" elicits visions of pasta, white bread, white potatoes, and cereals. Most people lump all carbohydrates into one big group that they believe will directly lead to obesity.

The Truth: Carbohydrates are your body's preferred energy source. Not all carbohydrates are the enemy; without them, you suffer from impaired brain functioning and fatigue. Foods that qualify as carbohydrates include grains (such as wheat, oats, rice, rye, and corn), fruits of all varieties, and vegetables of all varieties. Many people are surprised to learn that fruits and veggies are considered carbohydrates, but a quick review of the nutritional content of an apple will show contents of 20 grams of carbohydrates and minimal protein and fat. Therefore, it is considered a carbohydrate.

Carbohydrates can be divided into two categories: Simple (think pasta, white bread, and white potatoes) and complex (think sweet potatoes, asparagus, apples, whole grains and berries). It's true that indulging in simple carbohydrates will cause you to put on weight because they rapidly release glucose (sugar) into your bloodstream. Your body compensates for this by releasing insulin from your pancreas, which also causes the liver to store excess sugar as fat. Eating an abundance of simple carbohydrates causes your body to release more energy than it can use and release insulin more quickly, signaling your body to store more fat, resulting in weight gain.

However, complex carbohydrates help to energize your body without widening your waistline. Complex carbohydrates are the "good carbs" and are made up of chains of simple sugars. They also contain fiber, which helps to slowly release glucose (sugar) into your blood and minimizes insulin spikes and consequential weight gain.

The Plan: You do not need to consume large amounts of carbohydrates for energy, and you should only consume moderate amounts of good, complex carbohydrates (unless you're doing endurance training, such as training for a marathon or a UFC fight). For consistent energy, it is best to incorporate sensible quantities of low starch/low sugar carbohydrates into your meals throughout the day. For example: have a spinach and egg omelet for breakfast, a small serving of berries with raw nuts or nut butter for a snack, followed by a wild salmon fillet with a side of lightly steamed asparagus for lunch. The protein and fat from the nuts, eggs, and fish help to further slow down the release of glucose, so that you receive a steady and sustained stream of energy throughout the day. A general rule of thumb to follow is to eat starchy complex carbohydrates such as sweet potatoes or whole grains after a workout or after any rigorous activity, as your body will need more energy to recover.

#3: Use Fat to Lose Fat

The Misconception: Americans have been indoctrinated to believe that the main cause of obesity, heart disease and being fat is simply consuming fat. Consumer advocates, medical institutions/professionals, and government institutions almost unanimously support the consumption of low-fat, reduced-fat, and fat-free foods as a healthy alternative to full-fat foods. A diet is considered low-fat if 30 percent or less total daily calories come from fat, and are generally coupled with low protein intake (around 15 percent is typical) and a very high intake of carbohydrates (sixty percent or more is usually considered "healthy" by low-fat diet gurus). This model is based on a 1976 Senate report. In planning our meals, we have learned to discipline ourselves and cut the fat out: Only eat skinless chicken. Only eat egg whites. Eat butter substitutes instead of real butter. Avoid fat at all costs in order to reduce risk of heart disease and high cholesterol. We are used to thinking that eating any kind of fat will make you fat, lead to chronic illnesses, and will work against you if you are trying to lose weight. We are also accustomed to considering saturated fat a particularly artery-clogging food.

The Truth: Take a look at the following:

- Harvard's School of Public Health conducted a study that monitored 235 older women with varying levels of arterial plaque buildup over a three year period. The study concluded that the women who ate the most saturated fat had the least progression of plaque buildup in their coronary arteries.[20]

- In an interview with noted lipids researcher Dr. Mary Enig, renowned biochemist Richard A. Passwater, Ph.D., stated, "The idea that saturated fats cause heart disease is completely wrong, but the statement has been 'published' so many times over the last three or more decades that it is very difficult to convince people otherwise unless they are willing to take the time to read and learn what... produced the anti-saturated fat agenda." [13]

- In his book *Coronary Heart Disease: The Dietary Sense and Nonsense* (Harry Ransom Humanities Research Center, 1993), Dr. George V. Mann, participating researcher in the Framingham study,[14] states, "the diet-heart hypothesis [suggesting that high intake of saturated fat and cholesterol leads to heart disease] has been repeatedly shown to be wrong, and yet, for complicated reasons of pride, profit and prejudice, the hypothesis continues to be exploited by scientists, fund-raising enterprises, food companies and even governmental agencies. The public is being deceived by the greatest health scam of the century."[15]

- Dr. William Castilli, Director of the Framingham Study, concluded in 1992 that "in Framingham, Massachusetts, the more saturated fat one ate, the more cholesterol one ate, the more calories one ate, the lower people's serum cholesterol...we found that the people who ate the most cholesterol, ate the most saturated fat, ate the most calories weighed the least and were the most physically active."[16]

- Dr. Laura A. Corr, Consultant Cardiologist, and Dr. M.F. Oliver of the National Heart and Lung Institute in London conducted a 1997 comprehensive review of all studies to-date that explored whether low-fat or low-cholesterol diets worked as a treatment for heart disease. They concluded the following: "The commonly-held belief that the best diet for prevention of coronary heart disease is a low saturated fat, low cholesterol diet is not supported by the available evidence from clinical trials. In primary preventions, such diets do not reduce the risk of myocardial infarction or coronary or all-cause mortality. Cost-benefit analyses of extensive primary prevention programs, which are at present vigorously supported by governments, health departments, and health educationalists, are urgently required... Similarly, diets focused exclusively on reduction of saturated fats and cholesterol are relatively ineffective for secondary prevention and should be abandoned. There may be other effective diets for secondary prevention of coronary heart disease but these are not yet sufficiently well-defined or adequately tested."[17]

- According to the USDA, Americans' fat consumption has consistently gone down over the last 20 years, while the American national rates of obesity have increased.[18]

For almost two decades, studies have concluded that low-fat diets do not prevent obesity, reduce body fat, or prevent heart diseases. If you want to lose weight, avoid overeating due to cravings, and nourish your body all at the same time, then you must add fat to your diet. Don't panic! It's a good thing!

How does fat work in the body? Fat doesn't make you fat—it helps you to burn fat. Just like carbohydrates, not all fat is made equal and there are different kinds of fats: saturated (mono) fats come from animals and some vegetable sources (coconut and palm oil), and unsaturated (poly) fats come from sources like olive oil and avocados. Your body is dependent on healthy sources of fat for adequate hormone production, healthy brain and nervous system activity, cell function, and digestion. When your body does not get the fat it needs, these functions are impaired and degenerative diseases, hormone issues, and digestive dysfunction can develop.

What kinds of fat are good, and how do they keep me healthy? As you remember, the body digests carbohydrates and turns them into fast-burning glucose that is either used immediately or stored as fat. We have all been warned not to eat animal fats because saturated fats raise cholesterol levels in the blood. Healthy saturated fat actually protects your heart from damage, helps you burn fat, and keeps your body performing in peak shape. The reason for this is that a small amount of saturated fat takes a while to digest, allowing you to feel fuller for much longer and keep your food consumption in check.

Fat also helps you to absorb certain vitamins and minerals during the digestive process. Vitamins A, D, E, and K are all fat-soluble vitamins and can only be absorbed in the presence of fat, which is why foods rich in vitamins A, D, E, and K (like eggs yolks, wild-caught salmon, avocados, whole milk and meat) naturally contain fat. The body needs these vitamins to feed the brain, heart, liver, lungs, bones, cells, nervous system, hormones, and the reproductive system. Monounsaturated (Omega 3 fats, like in olive oil) and polyunsaturated fats are also great for heart health and for stabilizing cholesterol levels.

In order to succeed in your weight-loss goals, you need to remember that low-fat diets do not work. Some fat is good, and if you're not eating the right kinds of fat, you're not only setting yourself up for failure through the consumption of unsatisfying food, but you're also not absorbing the nutrients necessary to be healthy. Not eating enough of the right kinds of fat can be dangerous and ineffective, and often results in long-term weight gain.

What kinds of fats are actually bad for me? Man-made, heavily processed, and chemically altered fats that are found in more processed foods are the types of fats that should be avoided at all costs. These are called trans-fats, and they harden and damage the arteries, raise LDL (bad cholesterol), and lower HDL (good cholesterol). Having a high LDL level is a leading risk factor for heart disease and arthrosclerosis. The most common form of trans-fat is hydrogenated oil found in many processed foods such as butter substitute spreads and margarines. The foundation of trans-fats is unsaturated oil from vegetables or fruit (like soybean, olive, canola oils), which always retain their liquid form even when refrigerated. These oils become spreadable when they are chemically altered through hydrogenation or partial hydrogenation. These processes transform oils into solids and semi-solids (butter substitutes) by adding hydrogen. The process of adding hydrogen to oils not only increases your cholesterol levels, but also makes the oil more difficult to digest. Hydrogenated fats also contribute to increased triglycerides, lipoprotein, and inflammation, which leads to a hardening of the arteries and can result in a stroke, diabetes, or heart-attacks.

The Plan: Whole foods, in their unprocessed forms, are nutrient-dense and can benefit your health and weight-loss efforts in significant ways. Start to eat the right kind of good fats, and cut out trans-fat. Examples of healthy fats are extra virgin olive oil, avocado, avocado oil, raw nuts, cod, liver, fish oil, and cold water, wild-caught fish, like salmon. If you see the words "hydrogenated" or "partially hydrogenated" listed in a food's ingredients, avoid it completely.

#4: Sugar is the Enemy

The Misconception: You've probably heard that your number one enemy is fat. Maybe you've heard the culprit is carbohydrates. Many people also believe that sugar intake is only an issue for diabetics or individuals that have a family history of developing diabetes.

The Truth: For people struggling with weight loss, the real issue is sugar intake—and it applies to everyone, not just diabetics. The bottom line is that the more insulin your body releases, the more fat your body stores. This has earned insulin the nickname "fat-storing hormone." Although many people think that insulin is a man-made chemical sometimes injected to regulate blood sugar in diabetics, the truth is that everyone's bodies naturally produce insulin. Insulin is secreted by the pancreas, along with digestive enzymes, in response to the presence of glucose (sugar), amino acids (from protein), and fatty acids. Insulin's job is to regulate the transfer of sugar into fat: it processes glucose, amino acids, and fatty acids and stores them as fat throughout the body to prevent our blood sugar from skyrocketing to dangerous levels. The cells that store energy as fat are called adipocytes. Adipocytes produce leptin, a protein hormone that signals for long-term energy storage. Consuming limited amounts of sugar means that limited fat will be stored, and that the leptin hormone level will not trigger the body to store energy or fat long-term. However, the consumption of large amounts of sugar causes insulin to store fat in adipocytes and produce excessive levels of leptin hormones, which trigger the brain to switch into starvation-response mode. When in starvation mode, the brain tells the body to consume more calories for energy storage and increases lethargy for energy conservation. The calories from increased eating go unused and are stored as fat. Therefore, the excess sugar intake literally causes your body to ensure that you *cannot* lose weight, because it thinks your life depends on storing it.

However, sugar content isn't always easy to identify: we all know that sweets such as cookies, candies, cakes, and pastries are obviously loaded with sugar and should be avoided as much as possible. But many people don't realize there are many forms of sugar and a lot of foods have hidden sugar lurking just below the surface. Processed sugar is added to thousands of foods on the supermarket shelves today and can be difficult to spot, placing it on food labels with nicknames like "high fructose corn syrup." Recently, high fructose corn syrup has been used to replace sugar in many packaged and processed foods including breads, burger buns, crackers, soft drinks, and fruit juices.

Sugar often appears in foods you might consider healthy. Natural oatmeal is low in sugar, and is a staple of a healthy diet. Yet the pre-packaged, flavored kind that most people eat has up to 15 grams of added sugar per packet! Let's consider another favorite: tomato sauce. Pre-packaged marinara is loaded with corn syrup because it thickens the sauce, and therefore makes it cheaper to produce. Just half a cup of packaged tomato sauce contains 10 grams of sugar. Most whole-wheat breads contain high fructose corn syrup, and many yogurts are loaded with sugar that will send your body almost instantly into fat-storing mode.

High fructose corn syrup is a *toxin*. Fructose is structured differently than sugar and cannot be metabolized properly in the body. The liver is the only organ that processes fructose and most of it turns directly into very-low-density lipoprotein (VLDL), which most of us just call fat. Fructose is sweeter than sugar, meaning that we should use less of it, but we actually use more. When one considers the calories in both sugar and fructose, we observe that thirty percent more of the fructose we consume ends up as fat. So a low-fat diet full of fructose is actually a high-fat diet. Sugar, especially fructose, turns into fat. Furthermore, fructose blocks our stomach's hunger hormone, which starts a vicious cycle: people do not feel full from fructose foods and consequentially eat more and more because they never feel full. Fructose is at the root of the rampant pandemic of obesity, type 2 diabetes, heart disease, and other chronic illnesses.

Now, you may be thinking to yourself, *doesn't fructose occur naturally in fruit*? Yes, it does. However, the natural antidote to sugar is fiber. Although an apple does have fructose, it's also loaded with fiber that allows the fructose to metabolize properly. By the way, did you know that most processed and packaged foods have had all the fiber removed to increase shelf life?

The Plan: Like we discussed, the presence of high levels of glucose in the blood causes insulin levels to increase, and insulin is a fat storing hormone. Lucky for us, the body also produces glucagon, a hormone that does just the opposite. Glucagon breaks down fat to provide the body with more energy. Just as insulin helps the body store fat, glucagon helps the body burn fat.

Glucagon is released into the blood stream after a protein rich meal. We're not talking pounds and pounds of meat; even one small portion of protein will foster the release of healthy glucagon in the body. The best way to keep insulin and glucagon in perfect harmony is by balancing each meal with a healthy serving of protein (meat, poultry, fish, eggs or nuts), carbohydrate (fruit or vegetable), and fat (coconut oil, olive oil, avocado)—which is the foundation of this book. Following this simple plan can keep your blood sugar stable throughout the day, and restrict the release of insulin into the blood stream. You'll notice your meals plans are centered around foods that do not contain processed, toxic sugars, which ensures healthy and delicious recipes to get you going in the right direction. When you're shopping on your own, make sure you read food labels before you buy, and avoid any foods that contain these words in the ingredients list:

- sucrose
- fructose
- glucose
- dextrose
- galactose
- lactose
- maltose

#5: Don't Milk It

The Misconception: Milk does a body good.

The Truth: Milk does a body good. How's that for confusing? Just like carbohydrates and fats, only some forms of dairy will help you achieve your weight loss goal. People first started drinking milk approximately 7,500 years ago in central Europe after the mass-consumption of grains began. As you recall from the discussion of our Paleolithic ancestors' diets, living things do best on the diet for which they were genetically adapted. This means that our bodies were not made to process dairy. We are the only species of animal that drinks the breast milk of a different animal. Furthermore, pasteurizing milk kills off valuable enzymes and vitamins and changes the amino acid content, which can negatively affect your health.

The Plan: When focusing on weight loss, I find that a lot of people greatly benefit from eliminating milk and dairy products from their eating regimen for an extended period of time—or even forever. I have had thousands of clients shocked at how incredible they feel after just a few days of eliminating milk and dairy products, and report increased energy, accelerated weight loss, and digestive discomfort eliminated. If you are not quite ready to give up milk, your best option is to make the switch to raw cow's milk. You can research local farms to see if this is a feasible option for you.

As you can see, there's a lot more to this eating business than just putting food in your mouth. Don't get overwhelmed! Your meal plans have done the work for you by ensuring that you get the right kind and right amount of good foods. These foods will that help your body function and reach a healthy weight, while avoiding the foods that sabotage your body. Let's take a look.

Meal Plans and Recipes

Believe it or not, right now, you know exactly how to lose weight and keep it off for good.

In this section I am going to give you the meal plans to follow to shed tons of fat, just like thousands of program members already have.

I know how challenging it can be to start any new healthy eating plan, so I've ensured that these meals are not just delicious, but EASY to follow as well.

You will see that I have provided for you…

7 Breakfast Choices

8 Snack Choices

8 Lunch/Dinner Choices (can be used interchangeably)

Here's how this works.

Every day you will choose

1 Breakfast

1 Lunch

1 Dinner

2 Snacks

I have done all of the math, measuring and hard work for you so you don't have to worry about anything but eating the delicious food that follows.

Look through all of the meal choices and choose your favorite ones. I have provided recipes with each meal. I have also given you the "Quick Alternative" for those who are pressed for time.

Here's an example of what a great day in your new world of delicious food would look like:

Breakfast – Apple Chicken Sausage Patties

Snack – Almond Butter and Banana

Lunch – Chicken Fajita Salad

Snack – Chocolate Macaroons

Dinner - Garlic & Onion Burger and Green Beans

That's just one delicious example, and you'll be thrilled to see all of the amazing foods waiting for you to try.

Breakfast Choices (Choose 1 each day)

Apple Chicken Sausage Patties

On the Run Blueberry Shake

Easy Berry Protein Smoothie

Kale, Mushroom, & Sausage Scramble

Lox Omelette

Scrambled Eggs With Avocado

Turkey, Spinach & Tomato Stack

Lunch/Dinner Choices (Choose 2 each day, 1 is for lunch, 1 is for dinner)

Baked Herb Salmon Over Asparagus

Beef Minestrone Soup

Chicken Fajita Salad

Coconut Chicken Tenders With Sauteed Zucchini

Garlic & Onion Burger And Green Beans

Honey & Lemon Chicken Breasts With Asparagus

Garlicky Balsamic Pork Tenderloin Over Spinach

Steak Balsamic Salad

Snack Choices (Choose 2 each day)

Almond Butter Fudge

Chocolate Macaroons

Easy Afternoon "Pick Me Up" Shake

Hard-Boiled Eggs, Cucumbers & Tomatoes

Jerky

Oysters & Carrots

Raw Almond Butter & Banana

Raw Almonds & Apple

On the Run Blueberry Shake

Ingredients

1/4 cup Thai Coconut milk
1/3 cup Water
1 scoop Next Fitness Evolution Protein Powder
2 cups Raw Baby Spinach
1/2 cup Blueberries
To Taste Stevia

Directions

Place All ingredients (in order listed) in a powerful mixer, such as a Vitamix. Blend until smooth and well-blended. Enjoy! Makes 1 serving.

Quick Alternative

Smoothie made with 1 scoop of Protein Powder, water, ice and 2 1/2 cups of fruits and veggies of your choice.

Breakfast

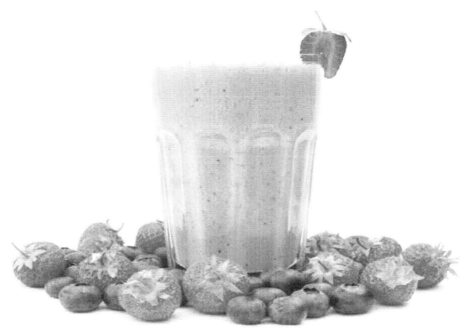

Apple Chicken Sausage Patties

Ingredients

1 Large Tart Apple (peeled and diced)
2 tsp Poultry Seasoning
1 tsp Sea Salt
1/4 tsp Pepper
1 lb Ground Chicken
1 tsp Coconut Oil

Quick Alternative

3 oz Ground Chicken (sautee in coconut oil and add salt and pepper) alongside 1 small apple

Directions

In a large bowl, combine the apple, poultry seasoning, salt and pepper. Break up the chicken over this and mix well. Shape into eight 3 inch patties.

In a large skillet with coconut oil, cook patties over medium high heat for 5-6 minutes on each side or until no longer pink. Drain any fat and enjoy! Makes 4 servings.

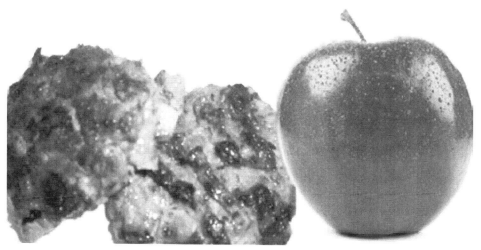

Kale, Mushroom & Sausage Scramble

Ingredients

2 Organic Eggs (beaten)
1/2 cup Mushrooms (sliced)
1/2 cup Kale (cut into thin strips)
1 oz Sausage (pork, chicken, turkey or beef)
1 tsp Raw Coconut Oil (for cooking)

Quick Alternative

2 Organic Hard Boiled Eggs
1 oz Cooked Sausage
1 cup Mushrooms and Kale sauteed in 1 tsp coconut oil

Directions

Melt coconut oil in medium skillet on medium-high. Saute mushrooms and sausage for 5-10 minutes (ensure sausage is cooked through). Add kale and saute until wilted. Add eggs. Season with unrefined sea salt and pepper. Stir frequently. Enjoy. Makes 1 serving.

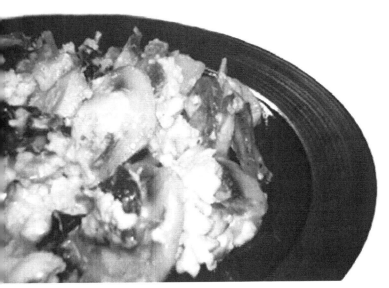

Easy Berry Protein Smoothie

Ingredients

1/4 cup Coconut Milk (full fat)
3/4 cup Water
1/2 cup Frozen Blueberries
1/2 cup Strawberries
1 scoop Next Fitness Evolution Protein Powder (vanilla)

Directions

Mix all ingredients in the blender until smooth. Enjoy! Makes 1 serving.

Quick Alternative

Mix coconut milk, water and protein in travel cup with lid. Shake vigorously. Enjoy alongside 1 cup of blueberries and strawberries.

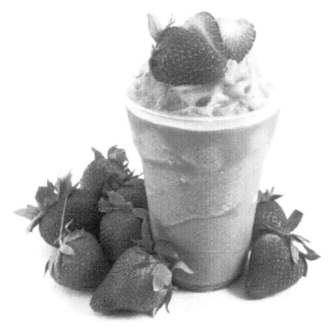

Scrambled Eggs with Avocado

Ingredients

2 Pastured Eggs
1 tsp Pastured Butter
1 Spring Onion (diced)
1/2 Small Avocado
To Taste Red Pepper Flakes
To Taste Salt and Pepper

Quick Alternative

2 Organic Hard Boiled Eggs served with 1/2 small avocado and seasoned with salt and pepper.

Directions

Crack eggs and whisk with a fork. Place butter in skillet. Once the butter is melted, add onions and cook until soft. Add eggs to skillet and season with salt and pepper. Sprinkle salt over avocado and serve with eggs. Makes 1 serving.

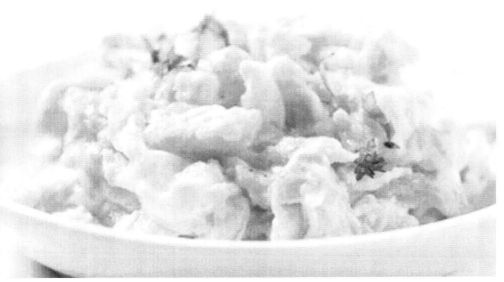

Lox Omelette

Ingredients

2 Large Eggs (whisked)
1 oz Smoked Lox
1 Tbsp Capers
2 Tbsp Red Onions (diced)
1 tsp Pastured Butter
1/2 tsp Fresh Dill (chopped)
To Taste Fresh Ground Pepper

Quick Alternative

Substitute 1 oz of cooked chicken or turkey (dark or white meat) instead of Lox.

Directions

In a small skillet over medium-high heat, melt butter. Once the butter has melted, add onions. Cook until onions are soft and translucent. Add capers and salmon for another 3-4 minutes. Pour eggs into the skillet on top of the fillings. Add fresh ground pepper. As the eggs cook, use a spatula and push the cooked eggs to the center of the pan. Tilt the pan forward and backward to let the uncooked eggs flow to the outer parts of the pan. Add 1/2 of the fresh dill. Fold the omelette over. Flip the omelette over and cook for another 45 seconds. Serve immediately and add remaining dill on top of the omelette. Makes 1 serving.

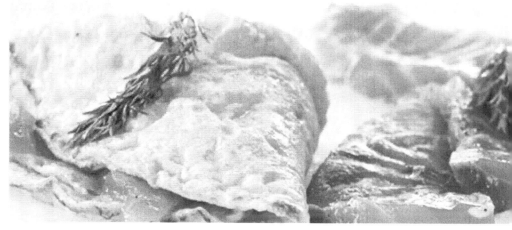

Beef Minestrone Soup

Ingredients

2 lbs Lean Organic Ground Beef or Ground Sirloin
1 cup Onion (chopped)
6 cups Water
1 cup Tomatoes (chopped)
1 cup Cabbage (shredded)
1 cup Carrots (chopped)
1/2 cup Celery (chopped)
1/2 tsp Dried Thyme
1 Bay Leaf
1/4 tsp Black Pepper
To Taste Sea Salt
5 tsp Grated Organic Parmesan Cheese

Directions

In a large heavy pan, cook beef and onion over medium heat until meat is no longer pink and onion is tender; drain off any fat. Add the water, tomatoes, cabbage, carrots, celery, thyme, bay leaf and pepper and salt; bring to a boil. Reduce the heat; cover and simmer for 1 hour. Discard bay leaf. Sprinkle each serving with 1/2 tsp of Parmesan Cheese (optional). Makes 8 servings.

Quick Alternative

3 oz Cooked Ground Beef
1-2 Tomato Slices
1 cup Celery and Carrots

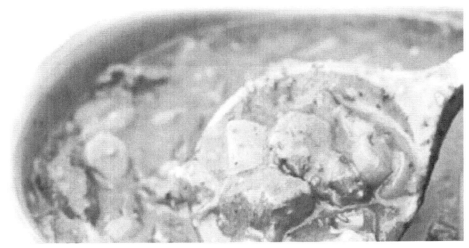

www.BeyondDiet.com

Baked Herb Salmon Over Asparagus

Ingredients

4 6-oz Salmon Fillets
1 Tbsp Olive Oil
2 Medium Garlic Cloves (coarsely chopped)
1/2 tsp Spike Vegetable Seasoning (or salt)
1 tsp Ground Cumin
1/2 tsp Freshly Ground Black Pepper
1 Tbsp Capers
1 cup Cilantro Leaves (coarsely chopped)
1 cup Flat-Leaf Italian Parsley (coarsely chopped)
2 tsp Lemon Zest
5 oz Fresh Lemon Juice
Makes 4 Servings

6 Medium Asparagus Spears
1 tsp Coconut Oil
To Taste Ground Cumin
Makes 1 Serving

Quick Alternative

6 oz Salmon Fillet (broiled)
6 Medium Asparagus cooked with 1 tsp coconut oil

Directions

Preheat oven to 350°F. Rinse salmon and place on lightly greased cookie sheet or in an ovenproof baking dish. Season with salt and pepper.
In food processor, process olive oil, garlic, Spike, cumin, pepper, capers, parsley, cilantro, lemon zeest, and lemon juice until well combined. Pour sauce over fish. Bake for 13-15 minutes, or until salmon flakes easily with a fork.

While the salmon is cooking, wash and dry the asparagus. Place in an oven proof baking dish. Pour 1 tsp melted coconut oil on asparagus. Salt and pepper to taste. Bake in the oven at 400°F for 12-15 minutes. Alternatively, I have cooked this in the oven at the same time as the salmon and it results in much crispier asparagus. Let it cook a bit longer than the salmon if you enjoy your asparagus a little softer.

Coconut Chicken Tenders with Sauteed Zucchini

Ingredients

1 1/2 lbs Chicken Breasts (cut in strips)
1 cup Dried Unsweetened Coconut (shredded)
1/2 cup Coconut Flour
1/2 tsp Sea Salt
1/4 tsp Ground Black Pepper
1/4 tsp Garlic Powder
1/4 tsp Paprika
1/3 cup Coconut Oil
1 Egg
6 Medium Zucchini
2 tsp Salt
2 Tbsp Butter
1/2 Lemon (juiced)
To Taste Salt and Pepper

Quick Alternative

4 oz Chicken Breast
1 cup Zucchini

Directions

Preheat oven to 400°F. Beat egg in a medium bowl. Mix coconut, flour, and spices in a separate flat pan. Dip chicken one at a time in egg, then dredge in coconut mixture making sure there is a nice thick coating. In a large skillet, heat coconut oil over medium-high heat. Place chicken strips in the oil and fry until browned on both sides. Transfer the strips to a cookie sheet and place in the oven. Cook until chicken is cooked through (about 5-7 minutes). Mix dijon mustard honey (2 parts mustard, 1 part honey) to dip!

Zucchini: slice into thin matchstick-like pieces. Add salt, stir well to mix, and let stand 1 hour. Rinse zucchini with water in a colander and squeeze dry in a tea towel. Melt butter slowly in a skillet over low heat. Raise heat to medium and saute zucchini for about 1 minute. Remove to a serving dish and season with lemon juice, salt, and pepper. Makes 6 servings.

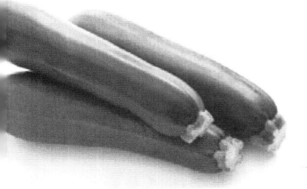

Chicken Fajita Salad

Ingredients

1 lb Chicken Breasts (sliced thin)
1 Tbsp Chili Powder
1 tsp Cumin
1/2 tsp Oregano
2 Garlic Cloves (chopped)
1 Red Onion (sliced)
1 Green Bell Pepper (sliced)
1 Red Bell Pepper (sliced)
To Taste Spinach and/or lettuce
1 Avocado
1/2 cup Salsa
2 Tbsp Coconut Oil

Quick Alternative

4 oz Cooked Chicken Breast over Salad (spinach or romaine lettuce, bell peppers, tomatoes, 1/4 avocado)

Directions

Cook bell peppers and onion until tender with 1 Tbsp coconut oil. Add in garlic for 1 minute. Remove from pan and set aside. Add 1 Tbsp more coconut oil and cook chicken for about 7-8 minutes over medium-high heat. Add in all spices and let simmer with a splash of water for 5 more minutes. Add back in veggies and lower heat and let simmer 5 more minutes. In a separate bowl, mix avocado and salsa. Arrange a bed of spinach or lettuce and top with chicken and veggies. Spoon avocado mixture on top and sprinkle with cheese. Makes 4 servings.

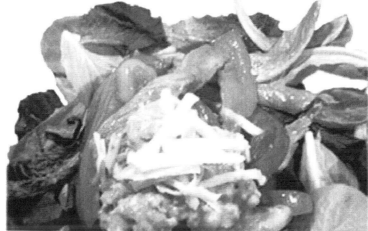

Honey & Lemon Chicken Breasts With Asparagus

Ingredients

4 Boneless, Skinless Chicken Breasts (about 4 oz each)
1 lb Asparagus (cut into pieces)
1/2 tsp Minced Garlic
2 Tbsp Raw Honey
1 tsp Lemon Peel (finely grated)
1 Tbsp Coconut Oil

Quick Alternative

3 oz Cooked Chicken Breast
1 cup Asparagus

Directions

Heat oil in large skillet over medium heat until hot. Add chicken breasts; cook about 5 minutes. Turn chicken over and add asparagus and garlic. Cook 1 minute or so, stirring occasionally. Add honey. Increase heat to medium-high; cover and cook 3-4 minutes or until chicken is fork tender, asparagus is crisp tender and juices are clear. Once done, stir in lemon peel. Makes 4 servings.

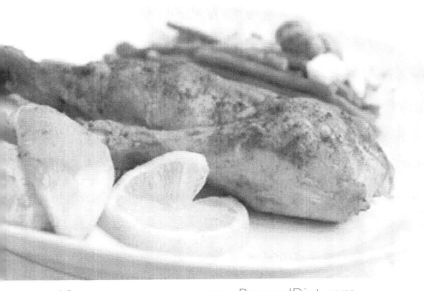

Garlic & Onion Burger And Green Beans

Ingredients

1 1/2 lbs Ground Beef
2 tsp Worcestershire Sauce
2 or 3 Garlic Cloves (minced)
3 Tbsp Onion (minced)
To Taste Salt
1 pinch Ground Black Pepper

3 lbs Fresh Green Beans
2 Tbsp Coconut Oil
To Taste Salt, Pepper & Garlic

Quick Alternative

3 oz Cooked Ground Beef
1 cup Green Beans

Directions

In a large bowl, mix together the beef, Worcestershire sauce, garlic, onion, salt, and black pepper. Combine the mixture well then refrigerate for 2 to 4 hours to allow the garlic flavor to infuse the meat. Form burgers into 4.5" thick patties. Grill or shallow fry for 6 minutes each side.

Green Beans: In large heavy skillet over high heat, stir-fry green beans and garlic in coconut oil until crisp tender. Reduce heat to medium, add pepper and salt. Cover and let steam for 2-3 minutes, stirring occasionally. Enjoy! Makes 6 servings.

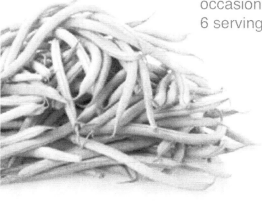
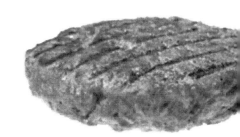

Steak Balsamic Salad

Ingredients

4 oz Flank Steak
5 Grape Tomatoes
1 cup Baby Arugula (or spinach)
1/4 cup Sliced Red Onion (or less to your liking)
1/2 Ripe Avocado, sliced into 2-3 long slices
To Taste Salt

Quick Alternative

4 oz Cooked Flank Steak, over 1/2 tomato (sliced) topped with 1/2 ripe avocado

Directions

Grill steak or cook in a skillet to desired temperature. Medium rare works well for this recipe. While it's cooking, mix the remaining ingredients to create the salad. Once steak is cooked, add on top of salad. Salt to taste. Makes 1 serving.

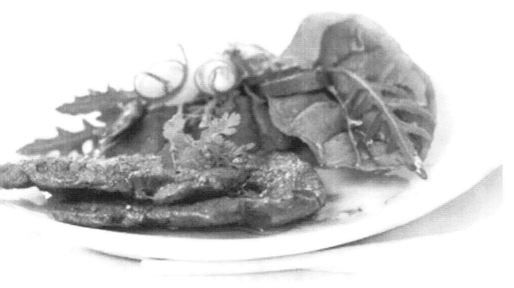

Garlicky Balsamic Pork Tenderloin Over Spinach

Ingredients

2 lb Pork Tenderloin (or 2-1lb tenderloins)
1/2 cup Extra Virgin Olive Oil
1/4 cup Balsamic Vinegar
1/2 tsp Pepper
1 tsp Unrefined Sea Salt
1 Tbsp Fresh Rosemary (finely chopped, if you don't have fresh, use dry)
1 Tbsp Fresh Oregano (finely chopped, if you don't have fresh, use dry)
1 Tbsp Fresh Thyme (finey chopped, if you don't have fresh, use dry)
5-10 Garlic Cloves (chopped; the amount depends on how garlicky you want these to be)
Makes 8 servings.

3 cups Fresh Spinach
1 tsp Coconut Oil
1 Garlic Clove (chopped)
Makes 1 serving.

Quick Alternative

4 oz Pork Loin broiled over sauteed spinach (in 1 tsp coconut oil)

Directions

In a medium bowl, whisk together garlic, oregano, thyme, rosemary, salt, pepper, balsamic vinegar, and olive oil. Cut excess fat off of the tenderloin and set in a deep dish. Pour the marinade over the top, flip the tenderloin around to coat, cover the dish and marinate in the refrigerator for at least 1 hour (and up to 24 hours).

Preheat oven to 375° F. Remove the tenderloin from the marinade and set in a roasting pan. Cover the pan and roast for 40 minutes, or until a meat thermometer reads 155° F. Remove from oven and let rest for 5-10 minutes before slicing.

Heat coconut oil in a pan over medium heat. Saute garlic for 5 minutes. Add in spinach and continue to sautee. Add unrefined sea salt to taste.

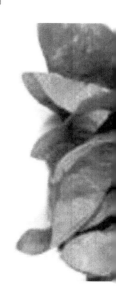

Almond Butter Fudge

Ingredients

2 cups Raw Creamy Almond Butter (unsalted)
1/2 cup Coconut Oil (warmed and softened so easily stirred)
3 Tbsp Raw Honey
1 tsp Unrefined Sea Salt
Optional: 1/2 cup Shredded Coconut

Directions

Mix all ingredients together in a medium sized bowl. Mix until smooth and creamy.

Line a square baking pan or dish with parchment paper. Put the fudge mixture into the pan and carefully smooth it out with a spatula. If it sticks to your spatula you can either dip it in water or coat the spatula with a bit of oil.

Freeze until solid, about aan hour. Remove the fudge by lifting the paper out of the pan. Place on a cutting board and cut the fudge into 16 equal pieces (approximately). Put them back into the pan, cover them really well and place them back into the freezer. This fudge can also be stored in the refrigerator in a tightly closed container. Serving size: 1 piece.

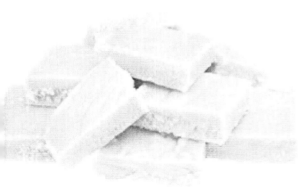

Turkey, Spinach & Tomato Stack

Ingredients

3 slices Turkey Bacon
1/2 cup Cooked Spinach
1/2 Tomato
1/2 Avocado
1 tsp Coconut Oil

Directions

Broil or bake bacon in the oven at 350° F. until crispy (about 15-20 minutes). Saute spinach in coconut oil. Slice tomato into 3 slices. Crumble bacon into smaller pieces. Layer a slice of tomato, spinach, avocado and crumbled bacon. Makes 1 serving.

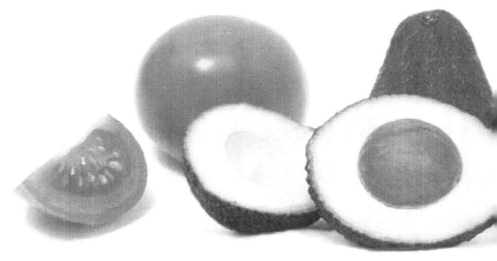

Snack

Easy Afternoon "Pick Me Up" Shake

Ingredients

1-2 cups Water (start with 1 cup and add based on consistency)
1 scoop Next Fitness Evolution Protein Powder
1/2 cup Frozen Blueberries or Strawberries
1 Tbsp Raw Honey

Directions

Add all ingredients in a blender (start with 1 cup of water and then add more to achieve desired consistency). Blend until smooth. Enjoy! Makes 1 serving.

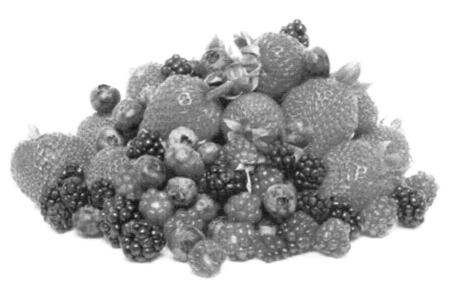

Chocolate Macaroons

Ingredients

1/2 cup Coconut Syrup
1/4 tsp Sea Salt
1/2 cup Coconut Flour
3 cups Organic Shredded Coconut
6 Large Organic Egg Whites

Directions

Place coconut flour, coconut and cocoa powder in a large bowl, mix well. Pour coconut syrup, eggs and sea salt into a double boiler. Whisk together until warm. Pour wet mixture into dry mixture. Mix well and put in refrigerator until hardened. Preheat oven to 325° F. Use a small ice cream scoop or melonballer to make little balls. Line on a cookie sheet. Bake for 15-20 minutes or until brown on the edges. Cool and enjoy! Makes 20 (serving size is 1 macaroon).

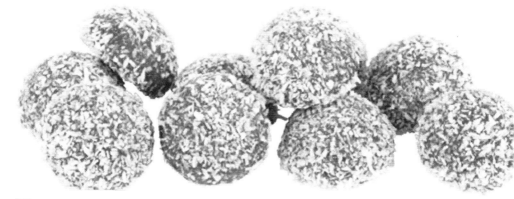

Jerky

Ingredients

2 oz Nitrate-Free Beef Jerky

~ or ~

2 oz Nitrate-Free Turkey Jcrky

Makes 1 serving.

Can be purchased from:
http://go.beyonddiet.com/grasslandbeef
or Whole Foods and Trader Joe's

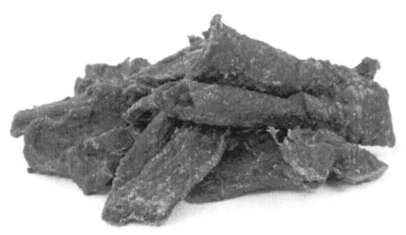

Hard-Boiled Eggs, Cucumbers & Tomatoes

Quantity

2 Hard-Boiled Eggs
1 cup Cucumbers & Tomatoes
To Taste Sea Salt

Directions

Chop cucumber and tomato for 1 cup serving. Slice each egg into half or quarter and place over veggies. Salt to taste. Makes 1 serving.

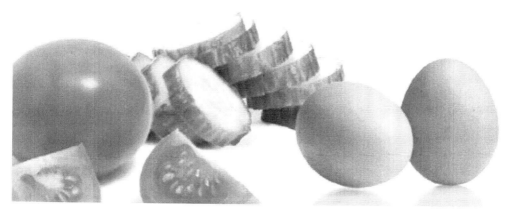

Raw Almond Butter & Banana

Quantity

2 Tbsp Raw Almond Butter
1/2 Small Banana

Makes 1 Serving.

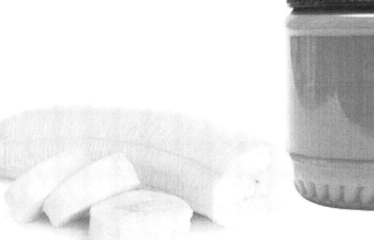
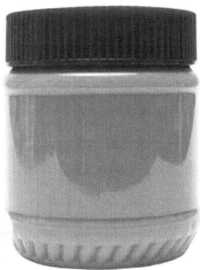

Oysters & Carrots

Quantity

1 can Crown Price Smoked Oysters
2 Large Raw Carrots (peeled)

Makes 1 Serving

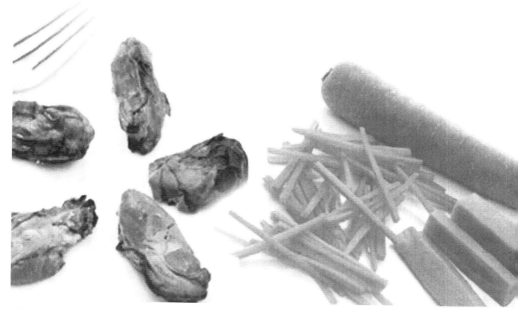

Raw Almonds & Apple

Quantity

1 oz Raw Almonds
1 Small Apple (any variety)

Makes 1 serving.

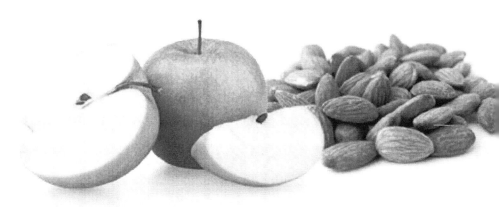

How To Shop The RIGHT Way

My job as your nutritionist and coach is to make this weight loss experience as simple as possible for you. That's why I've put together this detailed shopping list. Once you go through this guide there will be no confusion regarding which foods to avoid and which fat-melting foods to purchase. Now you'll always know exactly how to stock up on the most delicious, healthy foods for your optimal meal plans.

In addition to telling you the best foods to purchase to get the best results, I will also share with you my personal favorites and the staple items I always keep in my home.

You will notice that there is one very consistent theme throughout this entire guide (and program): NATURAL is always BEST!

I promise I am not going to suggest you solely eat nuts and berries or run out into the wilderness to find your food. That said, the easiest, fastest, and healthiest way to drop fat is to keep your food sources natural and free of chemicals, pesticides, hormones and additives.

Remember, if *and only if* it's natural—that is, it exists in nature—eat it. In other words, if a food contains ingredients that you can't pronounce or define, steer clear.

Natural foods span all the food groups and include fresh, unprocessed fruits and vegetables, unroasted nuts, whole seeds and grains, and unadulterated fats, dairy, and meat products. Foods in the artificial category include packaged foods, frozen meals, cookies and cakes, artificial sweeteners (e.g., saccharin [Sweet'N Low], aspartame [NutraSweet], and sucralose [Splenda]), hydrogenated oils (e.g., margarine and Crisco), and high-fructose corn syrup.

To understand why this distinction is important, you must understand the function of the liver.

The liver is the body's largest internal organ, and it's responsible for an astonishing variety of life-sustaining and health-promoting tasks, including those that make healthy weight loss and weight management possible. The liver is integral to countless metabolic processes, supports the digestive system, controls blood sugar, and regulates fat storage. One of the liver's most important functions—and the one most crucial to weight loss—is the chemical breakdown of everything that enters your body.

It is the liver's job to distinguish between the nutrients to be absorbed and the dangerous/unnecessary substances to be filtered out of the bloodstream. But when overwhelmed with toxins (like artificial sweeteners and other chemicals that are added to packaged foods), the liver gets "clogged" and cannot effectively process nutrients and fats. If your liver cannot process the nutrients and fats that your body needs, you will gain weight and you won't be able to lose it.

The liver also produces bile, a substance crucial to the detoxification of the body. Bile helps break down fats and assimilate fat-soluble vitamins. But when bile becomes overly congested with the toxins it's trying to filter out, it simply can't function properly. It becomes thick, viscous, and highly inefficient.

Anything that your body does not recognize as a food source qualifies as a toxin. Artificial sweeteners, for example, have zero calories because the body does not recognize them as food sources. But they still have to pass through the liver, as do other synthetic ingredients that you probably couldn't even pronounce.

Food-processing chemicals and other toxins also irritate the gastrointestinal system, and may cause bloating, constipation or gas in many people. Chronic constipation may also lead to difficulty losing weight, among other things.

Toxins are stored in fat cells—that is, they are embedded in body fat. The more fat in your body, the more toxins you can store. Stored toxins cause your cells and organs to become sluggish and inefficient. Toxins also attack and destroy cells and gene structures. They create an acidic environment in the body that is vulnerable to fungi, bacteria, parasites, worms, viruses, and many other pathogens. Organs and body systems under a toxic load lose their ability to metabolize and process fat effectively.

The body stores toxins in fat tissue. In fact, toxin storage is one of the main functions of fat stores; this protective mechanism keeps toxins away from vital organs. When you ingest fewer toxins, your body will not need as much fat to store them and will quickly begin to let go of excess fat. This process leads to the right kind of weight loss (from fat), as well as a healthy, disease-free body.

The body also stores toxins wherever it is weak. This makes the weak area even weaker and eventually can cause a cyst or disease. An area left diseased for too long becomes difficult to repair. To achieve an ideal weight and healthy body, it is vital to eat only clean, unprocessed food. From this point forward that is what I am going to help you do.

Throughout this guide, I mention specific product brands. I have researched these brands and personally recommend them based on their effectiveness and their fit within the program. If you cannot find these brands in person or order them online, you can make substitutions using your judgment and the principles you've learned here. However, I strongly recommend you use these brands, as I have already determined they deliver on their promises.

This guide will also help to explain the direct impact nutrition has on your health and weight loss. My goal is for you to become slimmer and healthier at the same time, because it's important to be just as fit on the inside as you are on the outside.

How would you like to lose weight and save money? My guide will teach you that quality, organic foods don't have to have to cost a fortune. I provide 20 money saving tips that'll help you save big at the register. After all, my goal is to trim your waistline, not your wallet.

Sound good? Well, let's get started.

The Best Way To Navigate The Supermarket

Wegmans, Harris Teeter, Shop Rite, Publix, Whole Foods and Trader Joe's all share the universal supermarket design. Upon entering any of these locations, you will quickly notice all perishable items (produce, meat, seafood, dairy and fresh baked breads) are located on the perimeter, or the edge of the store.

The perimeters are where you should spend at least 90% of your time. Why? Perishable foods are unprocessed whole foods and, therefore, have the most nutrients and minerals. These are the foods that will bring you the most success on this plan.

Let's start with produce....

Produce

We all know that fruits and veggies are good for our health, but what many people don't realize is that weight loss can be accelerated or slowed by how you choose your produce. Specifically I'm talking about the pesticides, herbicides and fungicides that may be added to your foods. These toxic chemicals overload your body (specifically your liver) and can create a "fat storing" environment in your body (exactly what you don't want when you're trying to lose weight!). So the less exposure you have to these harmful pesticides, the faster you will experience weight loss results.

Your *best* (and sometimes cheapest) *choice* for produce is LOCAL produce.

Yes, organic food is important (and we'll get to that in just a second), but many local farms grow their produce without synthetic pesticides, and can't afford the USDA organic certification, so these foods are less expensive.

Why is local produce cheaper? Well, when farmers grow produce on nearby farms, it costs much less to transport these foods to the local grocery stores. The farmers can pass that savings directly onto you in the form of lower prices. Local produce also has more nutrients than non-local produce. You see, when produce is harvested, it begins to lose valuable nutrients and antioxidants. Some produce can take several days or weeks before it even reaches the store! That means a lot of lost nutrients. So, how do decreased antioxidants impact your weight loss? Think back to earlier when I discussed how your liver works to filter out toxins in order to help you process and burn fat. The antioxidants in the produce help to neutralize these toxins in your body. Less toxins in your system means your liver won't have to work as hard to filter out impurities, giving it more time to help you burn more fat!

Local produce is sometimes the freshest produce available, and you'll feel good knowing you're supporting your local economy and your local farmer. The easiest way to find local produce is to seek out local farmer's markets in your area. A great resource to find one close to you is localharvest.org.

Organic is your *next best choice*. If organics are difficult to source in your area, focus on purchasing the regular variety foods with the lowest pesticide amounts. Remember, fewer pesticides equal greater fat loss.

I know you are probably thinking that organic produce costs 2-3 times more than regular produce. Actually, the cost of organic produce is a lot less than you may think. Organic produce is more available than it's ever been – you can even find it at Wal-Mart or Costco! I'll elaborate more on that later.

Did you know that certain fruits and veggies have more pesticides than others? This means that you don't *have* to buy all of your produce organic (unless you want to), so you'll spend less.

Here is an easy list to keep handy to help you decide which items to purchase organic:

Highest Levels of Pesticide Residue – should be purchased ORGANIC:

- Fruits
- Peaches
- Apples
- Strawberries
- Nectarines
- Pears

- Cherries
- Raspberries
- Grapes

Vegetables

- Spinach
- Bell/Hot Peppers
- Celery
- Potatoes

Lower in Pesticide residue - can be purchased CONVENTIONAL if necessary:

Fruits

- Pineapples
- Plantains
- Mangoes
- Bananas
- Watermelon
- Plums
- Kiwi Fruit
- Blueberries
- Papaya
- Grapefruit
- Avocado

Vegetables

- Cauliflower
- Brussels sprouts
- Asparagus
- Radishes
- Broccoli
- Onions

- Okra
- Cabbage
- Eggplant

Remember, you want to lower your overall exposure to pesticides and chemicals because these substances interfere with your liver function. Too many toxins will overload your liver, causing it to become sluggish, which means you'll burn fat at a much slower rate. These chemicals can also stay in your system for many years, long after your body has digested the food. These toxins can cause inflammation and increase your risk of developing certain cancers.

Pesticides do more than impair your weight loss – they also cause inflammation. Inflammation is the word we use to describe the situation when a specific part of your body has become swollen and causes you pain. Look carefully at the spelling and you'll see a familiar word – "flame." If you touched a hot oven and burned your hand, it would swell and cause pain. Well, think about inflammation as an internal oven. Your body is heating up on the inside and eventually inflammation will occur, and can cause a whole host of conditions such as arthritis and back pain.

If you have a minor burn, the pain and swelling goes away in a day or two. Can you imagine if your hand stayed swollen and uncomfortable for weeks, months or even years? It's hard to imagine your body's internal swelling, but that's what is happening. Weight loss helps to lower inflammation within your body. Buying cheaper, non-organic produce may save you a few dollars and cents in the short term, but you may be adding more fat and pain to your life in the long term.

Seafood

Seafood is a wonderful source of protein, when sourced correctly. Wild caught seafood is the only seafood I recommend. Farm-raised seafood is often loaded with high levels of polychlorinated biphenyl (PCB) and artificially colored using canthaxanthin and synthetic astaxanthin, which is not fit for human consumption.

In the same way that high levels of pesticides will affect your liver and negatively affect your weight loss, toxic chemicals found in farm-raised foods will also disrupt your body's natural ability to lose fat. Even worse, these chemicals have been shown to impair your thyroid, which makes fat loss even more challenging. Let me explain:

Farmed salmon contains 5 to 10 times the PCBs of wild salmon, according to an analysis conducted by the Environmental Working Group (EWG)[21]

A research study conducted by the Graduate Center for Nutritional Sciences at the University of Kentucky determined that PCBs encourage new fat cells to grow and increase inflammation. The study focuses on one PCB in particular, PCB 77. Researchers concluded that increased levels of this PCB promote obesity and heart disease. [21A]

The good news is wild caught salmon contain lower levels of PCBs and higher levels of Omega 3's. Omega 3's are crucial for heart health, and are also awesome for fat loss. Wild caught salmon feeds your heart and liver with these high quality fats. When you treat your liver and heart well, they reward you with a healthier heart and increased metabolism, so you burn more fat.

Farmed fish are fattened up with fishmeal, which contains plant material. Wild salmon eat smaller fish and krill, marine organisms that are rich in Omega 3's and give salmon their reddish-pink coloring. The plant material in fishmeal lowers the Omega 3 levels of farmed fish. Fewer Omega 3's mean less fat burning capability and less heart protection. According to a USA Today online article, both Dr. Andrew Weil, a respected medical expert, and The American Journal of Clinical Nutrition believe "farmed salmon have two to three times fewer Omega 3's than their wild counterparts." [22]

Wild caught salmon is a wonderful source of iodine; iodine helps the thyroid to function at its best. What does your thyroid have to do with weight loss? The thyroid is a major gland in your body. Think of it as your body's internal thermometer. **If your thyroid isn't functioning properly, you will burn calories and fat at a lower rate.**

Please adhere to the following guidelines when purchasing seafood:

1. Only purchase WILD CAUGHT seafood. Avoid FARM RAISED seafood.

2. Consume seafood with low mercury levels, such as salmon, cod and herring. Fish with HIGH mercury levels should only be eaten on occasion (tuna, swordfish and shark).

3. If you cannot get fresh wild seafood, your next best option is frozen wild seafood.

4. Another good choice (and very cost efficient) is wild caught canned seafood.

Some great sources for quality seafood are:

1. Vital Choice

2. Crown Prince brand (available at most supermarkets and on Amazon.com)

3. Wild caught frozen seafood – Trader Joe's, Whole Foods, and most supermarkets (Make sure it says WILD on the label.)

Fish LOW in mercury and safe to eat often:

1. Shrimp

2. Sardines

3. Tilapia

4. Oysters and Mussels

5. Clams

6. Scallops

7. Salmon

8. Crayfish

9. Freshwater trout

Fish HIGH in mercury and should only be eaten very occasionally:

1. Canned albacore tuna

2. Spanish mackerel

3. Fresh/frozen tuna

4. Grouper

5. Marlin

6. Orange roughly

7. Swordfish

8. Shark

Meats

When you are in the meat aisle, make sure to read the labels on the meat very carefully. The *best choice* for meats fits the following criteria:

- Organic
- Free-range
- Grass fed (pastured)
- Antibiotic free
- Hormone free

Why antibiotic and hormone free? Animals are routinely given growth hormones to make them bigger, so they produce more meat. Feedlot cattle are kept in pens where they are living on top of each other. In these types of unsanitary conditions, cattle often become sick; in order to combat this, cattle are given antibiotics. The result is that you ingest these dangerous antibiotics and hormones when you ingest the animal. This can undoubtedly lead to a long list of health problems including hormone disruption and increased fat storage.

If this isn't bad enough, cow are fed food that is designed to make them "fat" (corn, soy, grains), instead of the grass they were designed to eat. This doesn't only make the animal fat; it makes you fat as well, since you will essentially be consuming everything that animal consumes.

Grain fed, feedlot cows have meat that is high in Omega 6's, which cause inflammation. Inflammation results from feeding a cow (or any animal) food that its body cannot process. Animals are no different than humans in this respect. When the cow is slaughtered and you eat the meat, all of that inflammation goes right into your body and your liver is left to filter out the antibiotics and hormones in the meat.

We've all heard of antibiotic resistant bacteria causing infections such as MRSA. What you may or may not have known, though, is that these bacteria may be the indirect result of the antibiotics being fed to livestock.

In addition to causing inflammation, antibiotic ridden meat can make you sick. The Department of Agriculture reported in 1999, 2001 and 2006 that over 80% of pig farms, feedlot cattle, and sheep receive antibiotics for reasons other than treating illness. Many of the antibiotics used on these animals are similar to the ones we take to prevent or reduce infection. When animals are exposed to low doses of antibiotics over a long period of time, they can develop resistance to these antibiotics, just like we can. Even if you aren't exposed to any bacteria from the meat, at the very least you'll still be ingesting the antibiotics that the animal ate. Over time, ingesting low levels of antibiotics will make you vulnerable to antibiotic resistant bacteria.[23]

Grain fed meat is a double whammy in slowing down your weight loss. Not only does it increase the potential for pain in your body, but added by-products clog the liver, slowing down your fat burning ability and lowering your immunity. Yikes.

Grass fed beef, on the other hand, has higher levels of Omega 3's and lower levels of Omega 6's. Healthy cows raised on grass are also anti-biotic and hormone free. So make sure when you eat beef, you're eating grass fed beef.

The *next best choices* for meats are those that are **organic, free-range, and free of antibiotics and hormones.**

A *good (and price conscious) choice* for meats is:

- Raised without the use of growth hormones **(hormone free)**
- Raised without the use of antibiotics **(antibiotic free)**

If you see the word "natural," don't be fooled. Natural does not represent livestock that have been raised without the use of hormones and antibiotics.

If you buy meats, such as bacon or cold cuts, always make sure that you purchase these items **nitrate-free.**

My favorite source for all my meat and poultry is US Wellness Meats. US Wellness is an amazing and convenient resource for mouthwatering, nutritious, organic, grass fed meats with zero hormones, antibiotics, or nitrates - delivered right to your door! Check your resource guide for links where you can browse through prime cuts of chicken, beef, pork, lamb and even buffalo.

Dairy

The right dairy can be *very healthy* if you buy it from the right source.

The *best choice* for dairy is raw, grass-fed dairy. Raw dairy (unpasteurized and un-homogenized) contains more Vitamins A, D, C and B than the pasteurized, homogenized variety.

What do these vitamins have to do with weight loss?

Vitamin A is a fat-soluble vitamin that helps keep your mucus membranes moist. It is an important tool in fighting against infection and improving overall health.

Vitamin D is a very important vitamin for losing weight. Low vitamin D levels are associated with impaired pancreas cell function, which leads to insulin resistance. (24)

Vitamin C is a powerful antioxidant that lowers inflammation, and as you know by now, increased inflammation causes weight gain.

B vitamins function as co-factors that help your body turn carbohydrates into energy. They give you more "get up and go" in your step, so you'll move around more and burn more calories.

Raw whole milk also contains high levels of CLA (more on this below) and Omega 3 in its butterfat. In other words, it contains fat that helps to dissolve your fat.

If you are interested in purchasing raw dairy or would like to read about the facts behind raw dairy, pasteurization and homogenization, please visit http://realmilk.com.

The *second best choice* is store bought pastured dairy that is antibiotic and hormone free. Brands like Organic Valley are available in many stores, and many of its dairy products (milk, cheese, heavy cream, butter) are from grass fed (pastured) cows.

Remember when I mentioned CLA earlier in this section? CLA is a fat that helps your body burn fat; more specifically, it helps to reduce your overall body fat and to increase lean body mass instead. [26]

High levels of this fat are naturally present in the fat of foods such as grass fed dairy and meats. Homogenization is the process of breaking apart the fat globules in the milk in order to keep the cream from separating from the milk. The process involves using high pressure to break apart the globules so that the milk doesn't separate. Homogenization weakens the naturally occurring fat in dairy, which weakens the CLA and its ability to help you to burn fat.

A *good choice* for dairy is organic, antibiotic and BGH free (bovine growth hormone) that is **not** ultra-homogenized. Horizon, an organic brand that is sold in supermarkets nationwide, meets this description.

The same antibiotics and hormones that pose a threat to your weight loss and overall health in feedlot meat are also present in the dairy of feedlot cows. For this reason, I would ask that you follow the guidelines for meat when making dairy purchases.

Eggs

The criteria for buying eggs are very similar to that for buying meats. The *best choice* for eggs is grass fed (pastured) free range eggs, preferably from a local farm. These eggs are taken from chickens allowed to freely graze on grass and bugs. The chickens are treated humanely, and the eggs taste better and contain higher vitamin amounts than their store bought counterparts. You can observe this visually in the deep, rich yellow orange color of the yolk.

The *second best choice* is organic eggs rich in Omega-3's (ideally free-range). These chickens are fed organic feed that has higher Omega 3 levels than standard eggs.

A *good choice* for eggs is organic free-range/cage free eggs. These eggs come from free range or cage-free chicken (chickens that spend some time outside of a cage) that are fed natural feed.

Breads

When choosing breads, fresh bread with the fewest preservatives is always best. Of course, you want it to taste good too, so I recommend breads made from organic sprouted grains as the *best choice* for breads. Sprouting begins the enzymatic action that starts to break down the gluten, which makes the wheat more easily digestible and better tolerated by people with gluten sensitivities. Gluten, a protein found in wheat and grains like barley and rye, can cause digestive upsets for many people and prevent them from losing weight. A tasty example of sprouted whole grain bread is *Food for Life's Ezekiel 4:9*. Ezekiel Bread is organic and comes in multiple varieties to fit your meal plan, such as Cinnamon Raisin Bread, English Muffins, Rolls, and Tortillas.

It's not necessary for you to buy this specific brand, but I highly recommend it. The important thing for you to do is closely read the ingredients of any bread that you buy. Look for sprouted grains and avoid artificial ingredients, high fructose corn syrup and hydrogenated oils.

Rice Bread

If you're unable to obtain sprouted grain bread, your second best choice is bread made from rice flour. These breads are gluten and wheat free and easy to digest. The first ingredient for this type of bread should be "Brown Rice Flour." If you can't find rice bread with brown rice flour on the label, rice flour is your next best option.

Spelt Bread

Spelt bread is a *good choice* if you can digest gluten, but have trouble with wheat. Spelt belongs to the wheat family and contains gluten but is easier to digest than wheat. Check to be sure that the first ingredient is "spelt flour."

Make sure to carefully read the label of your bread to ensure that it does NOT contain the following ingredients:

- Hydrogenated Oil
- High Fructose Corn Syrup
- Bleached, enriched flour
- Wheat Gluten
- Artificial Flavor
- Sugars or Artificial Sweeteners (Aspartame or Sucralose).

Salt

Contrary to popular belief, some salt is actually healthy and delicious. Healthy salts are *unrefined* and untouched. It's important that you only purchase salt that states that it is unrefined. You can easily identify unrefined sea salt because of its unique color; natural sea salts come in all colors ranging from grey to black. One example is Celtic sea salt. This salt is a light grey color because it's unprocessed. It's dried naturally by the sun and wind. The lack of processing ensures the presence of all 82 vital trace minerals needed for optimum biological health and cell function.

Why is unprocessed sea salt essential to overall health and weight loss?

Unrefined sea salt still tastes of the sea – and that's a good thing. Its potent taste means you'll use less of the product than you would refined salt. The 82 trace minerals in unrefined sea salt have the same mineral content as blood plasma, meaning this salt is beneficial to your blood pressure. Unrefined sea salt contains low levels of calcium, potassium and magnesium, which are very important for stabilizing blood pressure. Table salt doesn't contain any of these three minerals.

Dr. Brownstein, M.D. supports the connection between mineral levels and blood pressure. He cites data from the National Health and Nutrition Examination Survey (NHANES) stating that "low mineral intake, specifically [of] magnesium, potassium and calcium were directly associated with high blood pressure."[25]

Salt also feeds your adrenals, the glands that sit on top of your kidneys. During times of stress, your adrenals release cortisol, the hormone that helps your body fight physical and emotional stress. Increased cortisol levels decrease your sensitivity to leptin, the hormone that makes you feel full, thereby increasing your chances of overeating.

Examples of recommended unprocessed sea salts are:

- Celtic Sea Salt (my favorite)
- Redmond's Real Salt
- Himalayan pink crystal salt

Regardless of which natural salt you include in your diet, make sure your salt does **NOT** contain any of the following:

- Sugar (added to stabilize Iodine and as anti-caking chemical)
- Aluminum silicate

Sweeteners

It's really no secret that sugar causes weight gain, disease and inability to lose fat. But some things just taste so much better with a little "sweet" to them, which is why it's great to know that there are many natural alternatives.

You are probably thinking to yourself, why do I need natural sugar alternatives? What's wrong with sugar free choices, like Equal or Splenda? Well, there's plenty wrong with those artificial sweeteners. In fact, the chemicals that these products contain are more harmful than sugar. Studies have linked artificial sweeteners to migraines, cancerous tumors and anxiety.

Did you know that chemical artificial sweeteners cause you to gain weight? A June 2010 issue of the *Yale Journal of Biology and Medicine* reveals that aspartame (NutraSweet, Equal), acesulfame potassium (Sunett or Ace K) and saccharin (Sweet N Low) increase your desire to eat more.

Below are some natural sweetener options that should be used in moderation:

Sweeteners Comparison Chart	Raw Honey	Brown Rice Syrup	Coconut Palm Sugar	Pure Maple Syrup (Grade B)	Stevia (Sugar Free)	Xylitol (Sugar Free)
Glycemic Index (GI) Rating	30	25	35	54	0	7
Available in powder and liquid form					✓	✓
Is minimally processed	✓	✓	✓	✓	✓	✓
Number of calories per serving (per teaspoon)	20	23	15	17	0	10
Contains trace minerals	✓	✓	✓	✓	✓	✓
Ideal for Cold Beverages			✓		✓ *	✓
Ideal for Baking and Hot Beverages	✓	✓	✓	✓	✓ **	✓

My everyday sweetener is stevia. I feel good knowing it is sugar free and plant based. Make sure your stevia product does NOT contain maltodextrin, dextrose, or any sugar derivative.

Some stevia powders include inulin fiber. This is fine because inulin fiber is a natural fiber found in fruits and vegetables. Still, make sure you monitor your own body's response as some have reported that their digestive system does not respond well to this kind of fiber.

I also like to use raw honey from time to time.

Honey, in its **raw and unrefined form**, contains a host of phytonutrients and enzymes that have a multitude of beneficial attributes. Refining honey uses heat, which destroys all of these enzymes and nutrients present in raw honey. Honey does not cause the rapid blood sugar rise and fall that white sugar does.

Oils/Fats

Forget everything you think you know about fats. This next section will cause you to re-think the role of fat in your diet. In this section I'll show you that saturated fats are good for you, certain fats have health benefits, and fats can even help you burn fat.

Yep, you read that correctly: saturated fats can be very good for weight loss and heart health! Many fats that you believe are bad for you - namely butter, chicken skin, coconut oil and whole fat dairy - are actually good for you. These are the same fats that our ancestors ate for thousands of years. So why have we given these exact same fats such a bad reputation over the past 70 years?

Before you decide I must be crazy, let me assure you that I can back up these statements with facts.

I am going to start off by explaining the term "cholesterol."

Inflammation, not cholesterol, is the enemy when it comes to your health. Your body needs cholesterol to perform properly. Cholesterol is a waxy substance found in your blood and in every cell in your body. It makes up the building blocks for hormone production and bile that help you to digest and burn fat. It is also necessary for proper brain growth.

Your liver is responsible for producing over 70% of your cholesterol. There are two types of cholesterol, HDL and LDL.

HDL is known as the "good cholesterol." This is the cholesterol that reduces or prevents the buildup of plaque in your arteries (also known as atherosclerosis).

LDL is known as the "bad cholesterol." This cholesterol is responsible for narrowing your arteries.

In 1953, scientist Ancel Keys conducted a study that led to the conclusion that consuming saturated fat leads to heart disease. In the experiment, scientists fed cholesterol to rabbits and saw a significant increase in atherosclerosis and heart attacks. They also saw that feeding rabbits with vegetable and seed oils, like sunflower oil, didn't cause atherosclerosis. Of course, there is major flaw in this study. Rabbits eat plants and they usually receive very little (if any) cholesterol in their diet. This is not true for humans. Furthermore, the scientists in this study fed oxidized (rancid) and altered saturated fats to these rabbits. Oxidized fats will raise the LDL of any organism because these fats are damaged and their protective qualities have been destroyed. Finally, Keys failed to address a significant amount of data when formulating his conclusions. He was presented with information comparing the saturated fat consumption and heart disease from 22 different countries. He only chose to focus on the information from 7 of these countries. These mistakes lead to his false conclusions.

The truth is oxidized vegetable oils were the real culprit in heart disease, not saturated fat. Naturally occurring saturated fats (like coconut oil, raw butter) are beneficial.

The following admission comes from Mr. Keys himself, more than 40 years after his original theory: "There's no connection whatsoever between the cholesterol in food and cholesterol in the blood. And we've known that all along. Cholesterol in the diet doesn't matter at all unless you happen to be a chicken or a rabbit."

Contrary to popular belief, saturated fats are also good for your heart. Harvard School of Public Health conducted a study that monitored 235 older women with varying levels of arterial plaque buildup over a three year period. The study concluded that women who ate the most saturated fat had the smallest progression of plaque buildup in their coronary arteries.[20]

In fact, there are studies that show increased rates of death when cholesterol levels are too low. According to the Framingham Study [14] which followed 15,000 participants over 30 years, "There is a direct association between falling cholesterol levels over the first 14 years and mortality over the following 18 years."

I recommend that you buy only virgin cold-pressed, unrefined oils (mainly olive and coconut). You should avoid all other vegetable oils (canola, soybean, etc.) – the average human diet contains way too much of these ingredients.

Olive oil is flavorful oil that is derived from olives. Organic olive oil is naturally pressed and has superior taste.

For medium-heat cooking (sautéing) and use straight from the bottle (on salads and cooked foods), choose organic **extra-virgin olive oil**. It should be cold-pressed, cloudy (unrefined), and sold in a dark bottle.

Virgin Coconut Oil

Coconut oil has a thermogenic effect on the body, which means that it helps you to burn fat. It's also a great energy booster!

The healthy saturated fats in coconut oil have anti-microbial properties that help keep gut flora (good bacteria) in check. Coconut oil also contains high amounts of lauric acid, which helps to keep your immune system strong against viruses like the flu.

Coconut oil **should** be:

- Organic
- Virgin
- Cold-pressed

This type of oil **should not** contain any chemicals (including hexane).

My personal recommendations for coconut oil are CocoPura and Nutiva. Both brands are cold-pressed, without the use of chemicals, and retain the smell and natural healing properties of coconuts.

Grass fed Butter

You should also use **butter** for cooking, in recipes, or on top of vegetables.

For high heat cooking, I recommend butter and virgin coconut oil.

Organic raw butter made from grass fed cows would be your *best choice*. If you are unable to find raw, organic grass fed butter, organic butter from grass fed cows is your *second best choice*. If either is not available, organic butter can also be used.

Make sure the ingredients on the label are:

- Organic cream (or milk)
- Salt (I purchased unsalted and then add my own Sea Salt.)

Food Staples

There are certain staples that you should always shop for. I highly recommend these foods for a successful fat loss meal plan.

1. Virgin Coconut Oil
2. Stevia
3. Organic Eggs (ideally pastured)

4. Organic Vegetables (To cut costs, remember to buy organic for produce listed on the "Dirty Dozen" list.) Examples: lettuce, peppers, zucchini, sweet potatoes

5. Organic Fruit (To cut costs, remember to buy organic for produce listed on the "Dirty Dozen" list.) Examples: Blueberries, apples, pears, strawberries, pineapple

6. Organic Meat and Poultry (All meats should ideally be grass fed and antibiotic and hormone free.) Examples: Bacon (nitrate free), Beef, Dark Chicken and Turkey

7. Sprouted Whole Grain (SWG) Bread - Look in the Freezer Section. (This is an optional staple. Only use this if you want to continue eating bread.)

8. Raw Nuts (Great for snacking!) Examples: raw almonds, walnuts and macadamia nuts

9. Unrefined Sea Salt (Celtic Sea Salt)

Oragnic On The Cheap: 19 Ways To Save Big Bucks On Organic Groceries

Quality costs more – but these days, everyone can benefit from saving money. Fortunately for you, there are numerous ways to save money at the grocery register. I've listed the top 20 resources. For added convenience, most of these resources are available within your own community (if you live in a city, you can also access many of these resources).

I care about all of my clients, and I want to do everything in my power to guarantee your success on your weight loss program. One of the easiest ways that I can do this is to help save you money so that you can lose weight and become healthier, without going broke.

1. Warehouse Shopping Costs

Warehouse discount clubs have long been appreciated by the public for saving money on bulk items like paper towels and toilet tissue. Now you can add organic items to that list. Many warehouse discount clubs, like Costco and BJ's, have a large selection of organic foods including meats, produce, dairy, eggs and soups.

Chances are you probably already have a membership to one of these clubs. If you don't, you can get twice the value for half the price by splitting the membership with a friend or family member. If you don't have a membership, another option is to go shopping with someone who does. When you've finished shopping, give the person with the membership the money for your portion of groceries!

If you live in a part of the country with a super Wal-Mart, be sure to check out their organic food and produce sections as well.

2. Farmer's markets – Farmer knows best

Farmer's markets are a great resource. The produce is local, the farmers are friendly, and the quality is outstanding. Many farmers don't use synthetic pesticides for their crops. Since crops are grown locally, they don't have to be transported far distances, which means your food won't lose valuable nutrients during shipping. Best of all, if you have a question about a particular item, you can always ask the source directly!

Because produce is local, farmer's market prices are generally cheaper than organic and conventional produce.

3. Community Supported Agriculture (CSA) – Produce delivered to your door

CSAs are a new way to bring the farm to your door. CSAs allow you pay for a membership to purchase a share from a local farm for a season. Every week you'll receive a box of seasonal produce. The CSAs will give you a list beforehand of the seasonal produce, so you know how much of each item you'll be receiving. Prices for the membership (over the course of the season) are usually much lower than purchasing these items at a supermarket. CSAs also offer other food items such as meats, dairy and homemade bread.

Not only is this option convenient, it's cost effective. If you are a single person, you can save even more money by splitting the membership (and groceries) with another friend.

4. Go Directly to the Farm

Going directly to the farm allows you to purchase the freshest cuts of meat available – directly from the source. It's also the best place to get the cheapest price per pound. When supermarkets buy meat, they pay for shipping, packaging, and the equipment to cool the meat. The store then passes these costs to you, the consumer. Buying the meat directly from the farmer allows you to bypass the middle-man so that you can save money.

Many local farms feed their livestock grass and their chickens natural feed, so your food will still be nutritionally dense – for much less! If you want to confirm what the animals are eating, you can ask the farmer these questions directly.

Ask your family, friends and people in your neighborhood if they would like to split up the meat of a cow, pig, chicken, or lamb. Let them know that they will most likely pay less per pound than going to the store – I'm sure you'll have no problem finding at least 10 willing participants.

Many of these farms give you the option to buy dairy directly from them as well.

5. Build Your Own Chicken Coop

As I've previously stated, pastured eggs are superior to conventional eggs in both nutrition and taste. If you live in the country you can make sure that you always have access to the freshest eggs around. How is this possible? By building your own chicken coop. You don't have to be an engineer to build a chicken coop; there are many do-it-yourself e-books that can show you how to build your own chicken coop, step by step.

6. Buy in Bulk Online

Buying meats in bulk is not something you can do only at the farm; you can also buy bulk quality meats online. Buying online allows you to split the costs of the food with your friends and neighbors, and have the meat delivered directly to you. This is a great option if you're busy and don't have time to drive to your nearest farm.

I recommend US Wellness for bulk quality meats.

7. Eat a Smaller Quantity of Processed Foods

This may seem like an obvious solution, but you'd be surprised by how much money you shell out on snacks and boxed foods. This is one of the easiest ways to save money on your grocery bill. You can test this option yourself: for 1 month buy ½ to a ¼ of the processed foods that you'd normally buy. At the end of the month, compare your previous month's bills with your bills for that month – guaranteed you'll see the difference.

8. Make more delicious meals at home, eat out less

Another easy way to save money is to make more of your meals at home, including lunches. On Sunday, set aside a few hours to cook your food for the week. Make about 6-8 simple meals, wrap them well and freeze them. Multiple meals allow you to rotate your meals, so you don't have to keep eating the same foods over and over again. Reward yourself by going out to dinner at your favorite restaurant at the end of the month. Bank the remainder of the money that you've saved.

9. Whole Nutrition = The Sum of all the Parts

Use all of the parts of the animal including the organs. Not only are these parts nutritionally dense, they're cheap! Make sure that the organs are from pastured (grass-fed) animals.

10. Is There A Butcher in the House?

Find a good quality butcher in your neighborhood for cheap bones and organs. Many people no longer make their own stocks, and many people do not eat organ meats. Butchers will most likely throw these items away. They'll probably sell these items to you for very little money. If you're lucky, they may even give them to you for free. Remember to request grass-fed bones and organ meats as they're the best choice.

11. Grow Your Own Veggies

One of the best ways to save money on produce is to grow your own at home. Growing your own garden is easier than you think. Many people have been doing this as a hobby for years. E-books make tending your own garden easier than ever before.

I highly recommend *"Food for Wealth"* – If you are new to the world of organic gardening, this book breaks down the art of growing your own produce into simple steps. Once you've mastered the basics, I recommend a second book, *"Aquaponics4you."* This book seriously improves your organic gardening techniques to yield more vegetables for your efforts. The combination will give you the best value for your home grown organic garden.

12. Co-ops

A food co-op is a collectively owned grocery store and a great central location for natural and organic foods. Co-op members often receive discounts on many items within the store. Many co-op memberships require you to work at the store for a few hours a month in exchange for a free membership!

13. Private Label Brands

Look for sensibly priced Private Label Brands (PLB) at your supermarket. 365 Everyday is Whole Foods' PLB. The ingredients are outstanding on most of their items and the price difference can be as much as $3-4 less than their brand label counterpart! In fact, all Whole Foods PLB items are natural, and most are organic!

14. Dairy You Can Make at Home

If you are an avid cook or feel particularly adventurous in the kitchen, you can really stretch your dollars and make your own grass-fed yogurt and butter from your pastured or raw milk.

15. Bake Your Own Bread

You can also make your own delicious, sprouted bread at home. For more money saving goodness, use this simple, yet hearty recipe.

Gluten Free Rice Bread Recipe

Ingredients:

1 cup brown rice

7/8 cup water

1 egg

1 teaspoon baking powder

1/4 teaspoon salt

Soak the rice in the water overnight (6-12 hours). Grind the rice and water mixture in blender until the rice particles in the batter reach the consistency of fine salt. Add egg, baking powder and salt to the batter. Mix well.

Bake COVERED for 30 minutes in a well-oiled eight-inch iron skillet or a casserole dish (a well-seasoned cast iron skillet can't be beat for baking with rice).

16. Freeze It

Buy fruits and vegetables in bulk, when they're in season. Double wrap the produce in freezer resistant wrapping, and place them in freezer bags to keep out freezer burn and lock in the flavor.

17. Bartering food with neighbors and friends

Save money on groceries by trading food items with your friends and neighbors in your community. This is also great if you have more food items than you or your family needs.

18. Online Coupons

You don't have to go searching your Sunday paper to clip coupons - unless you want to.

19. Have a Potluck Dinner!

This is the easiest and most social way to save money. Once a week (or however often you choose), have a healthy potluck dinner with your family, friends and neighbors using organic foods. Assign one or two dishes to each person. For the price of two side dishes, you'll have access to a full banquet of delicious, nutritious food!

Well there you have it, a comprehensive guide that will help you save money, while achieving weight loss success.

I hope that you have enjoyed this guide as much as I've enjoyed creating it. Please take this guide with you whenever you go shopping.

Here's to Your Weight Loss Success!

Happy Shopping and Saving!

Use the QR code below or visit
www.MyFatBurningBonus.com
and get your FREE Mouth Watering Recipes and more!

References:

(1) The Paleo Diet.. Loren Cordain, Ph.D. 2010 Loren Cordain, Ph.D.,

(2-12) From the Mid America Heart Institute, Cardiovascular Consultants, Kansas City, Mo (J.H.O.); and Department of Health and Exercise Science, Colorado State University, Fort Collins (L.C.).: And Dr. Loren Cordain, Ph.D. of the Department of Health and Exercise Science at Colorado State University. 2004.
http://thepaleodiet.com/wp-content/uploads/2011/02/Cardiovascular-Disease-Resulting-From-a-Diet-and-Lifestyle-at-Odds-With-Our-Paleolithic-Genome-How-to-Become-a-21st-Century-Hunter-Gathererabstract.pdf

(13) Dr. Mary Enig, Consulting Editor to the Journal of the American College of Nutrition, President of the Maryland Nutritionists Association, and noted lipids researcher.
http://www.drpasswater.com/nutrition_library/enig1_interview.html

(14) The Framingham Heart Study is a long-term, ongoing cardiovascular study on residents of the town of Framingham, Massachusetts.
http://www.framinghamheartstudy.org/index.html

(15) Dr. George V.Mann, participating researcher in the Framingham study and author of CORONARY HEART DISEASE: THE DIETARY SENSE AND NONSENSE, Janus Publishing, 1993.

(16) Dr. William Castilli, Director of the Framingham Study. Archives of Internal Medicine, 1992.

(17) European Heart Journal, Volume 18, January 1997.

(18) Robert H. Lustig, MD. Professor of Clinical Pediatrics, in the Division of Endocrinology Director of the Weight Assessment for Teen and Child Health (WATCH) Program at UCSF. UCSF's Lustig Discusses the Role of Fructose in Pediatric Obesity. August 12 2006

(19) Beyond Diet.
http://www.beyonddiet.com/Members/Pages/AboutIsabel

(20) Web MD. Salynn Boyles. December 8, 2004.
http://www.webmd.com/heart-disease/news/20041208/are-saturated-fats-heart-healthy

(21) Nutrition Research Center. Farm Raised Fish Not So Safe. March 20, 2008
http://www.nutritionresearchcenter.org/healthnews/farm-http://www.nutritionresearchcenter.org/healthnews/farm-raised-fish-not-so-safe/

(21A) Arsenescu V, Arsenescu RI, King V, Swanson H, Cassis LA.Polychlorinated biphenyl-77 induces adipocyte differentiation and proinflammatory adipokines and promotes obesity and atherosclerosis. Environ Health Perspective 2008 June 116(6):761-8. Graduate Center for Nutritional Sciences, University of Kentucky, Lexington, KY 40536, USA.

(22) USA Today. Nick Jans. June 10, 2002.
http://www.usatoday.com/news/opinion/editorials/2002-10-06-oplede_x.htm

(23) Center for Global Development. Kammerle Schneider & Laurie Garrett, Council on Foreign Relations. June 19, 2009. http://www.cgdev.org/content/article/detail/1422307

(24) Live Strong. Cydney Walker. March 5, 2011.
http://www.livestrong.com/article/397284-vitamins-herbs-to-treat-insulin-resistance/#ixzz1sEK5EPre

(25) A Grain of Salt. Dr. David Brownstein, MD. Salt Your Way To Health. 2006
http://celticseasalt.com/PDF/BrownsteinSaltArticle.pdf

(26) Whigham LD, Satter CA, Scholler DA (2007). "Efficacy of conjugated linoleic acid for reducing fat mass: a meta-analysis in humans. Am". J Clin Nutr 85 (5): 1203–1200

Notes:

Notes:

Visit www.MyFatBurningBonus.com And Get Your FREE
Mouth Watering Recipes And More!

Notes:

Notes:

Notes:

Notes:

Notes:

Notes:

Visit www.MyFatBurningBonus.com And Get Your FREE
Mouth Watering Recipes And More!

Notes:

Made in the USA
San Bernardino, CA
01 May 2014